MEDICAL DEVICE USE ERROR

ROOT

CAUSE

ANALYSIS

MEDICAL DEVICE USE ERROR

ROOT

CAUSE

ANALYSIS

Michael Wiklund
Andrea Dwyer
Erin Davis

Illustrations by Jonathan Kendler

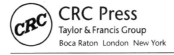

CRC Press
Taylor & Francis Group
Boca Raton London New York

CRC Press is an imprint of the
Taylor & Francis Group, an **informa** business

CRC Press
Taylor & Francis Group
6000 Broken Sound Parkway NW, Suite 300
Boca Raton, FL 33487-2742

Printed on acid-free paper
Version Date: 20151020

International Standard Book Number-13: 978-1-4987-0579-0 (Hardback)

This book contains information obtained from authentic and highly regarded sources. Reasonable efforts have been made to publish reliable data and information, but the author and publisher cannot assume responsibility for the validity of all materials or the consequences of their use. The authors and publishers have attempted to trace the copyright holders of all material reproduced in this publication and apologize to copyright holders if permission to publish in this form has not been obtained. If any copyright material has not been acknowledged please write and let us know so we may rectify in any future reprint.

Library of Congress Cataloging-in-Publication Data

Names: Wiklund, Michael E., author. | Dwyer, Andrea M., author. | Davis, Erin, author.
Title: Medical device use error : root cause analysis / Michael Wiklund, Andrea Dwyer, and Erin Davis.
Description: Boca Raton : Taylor & Francis, 2016. | Includes bibliographical references and index.
Identifiers: LCCN 2015021867 | ISBN 9781498705790 (hardcover : alk. paper)
Subjects: | MESH: Equipment Failure Analysis. | Root Cause Analysis. | Equipment Design--methods. | Medical Errors--prevention & control.
Classification: LCC R729.8 | NLM W 26 | DDC 610.289--dc23
LC record available at http://lccn.loc.gov/2015021867

Visit the Taylor & Francis Web site at
http://www.taylorandfrancis.com

and the CRC Press Web site at
http://www.crcpress.com

Contents

Foreword

This is the latest book in a series of usability-related texts from Michael Wiklund and colleagues that has focused on human factors engineering of medical devices. In this newest contribution to the series, titled *Medical Device Use Error: Root Cause Analysis,* Michael Wiklund, Andrea Dwyer, and Erin Davis address the very important safety topic of analyzing use errors. They provide excellent, practical guidance on how to methodically discover and explain the root cause of a use error—a mistake—that occurs when someone uses a medical device.

This newest book complements Michael Wiklund and colleagues' previous books: *Usability Testing of Medical Devices, Handbook of Human Factors in Medical Device Design, Designing Usability into Medical Products, Medical Device and Equipment Design,* and *Usability in Practice.*

Readers familiar with the application of human factors engineering ("HFE," also called usability engineering) to medical devices will no doubt appreciate that regulators of medical products have for the last 10 years used the term "use error," as opposed to the more common, but somewhat inaccurate, terms "human error" or "user error." The contemporary term "use error" is neutral regarding the cause. It does not automatically blame the user, as implied by the previously used term "user error." Philosophically consistent with using the contemporary term, root cause analyses should assess all possible causes of use error, and doing so is what this book prescribes. It calls on readers to view and access use errors with the same attitude and rigor that they would apply to an electrical defect, such as a short circuit producing a leakage current, that could shock a user. Note that device developers do not blame users for shocks due to poor electrical insulation or grounding, and neither should they blame users for pressing the wrong button because it is poorly labeled or an array of buttons are too closely spaced, for example.

In the broader scheme, manufacturers and medical product designers should strive to design a device that does not induce usability-related errors during interaction with the device's user interface, now widely known as use errors. The designer should not blame the user for failing to read the instructions or not learning to use the device during training. Instead, as described in this book, the designer should focus on whether the root cause of the problems might be due to user interface design flaws or other usability defects, such as poor navigation, misleading function labels, confusing symbols, difficult-to-use controls, illegible displays, or poorly communicated error messages. Thus, the term "use error," by its very nature, calls for an investigation of why the use problem exists, and this is best done through root cause analysis. As director of human factors engineering at AbbVie (formerly part of Abbott Laboratories), I have considered it very important to make sure that product developers understand and support such analyses because it is the path toward essential insights into optimizing user interactions with medical devices as well as other equipment, such as laboratory instruments.

After working for three decades in the human factors engineering business, I have a deepening appreciation for the history behind our current methods, so indulge me as I share some history related to the book's topic. The method of root cause analysis has been around for a long time and has been a major component in business excellence tool kits, such as Six Sigma and Lean. In the 1950s, Sakichi Toyoda introduced the term in Japan at what is now the Toyota automobile company. Toyoda-san promoted the concept of "Five Whys," which called on investigators to ask "why" five times to get to the heart of a problem. This is how one might start with a car problem, such as a seized engine, and trace it back to inadequate oil, a difficult-to-access dip stick, and the lack of an oil pressure gauge.

I am sure that root cause analyses, including asking a lot of "whys," have helped Toyota isolate and remedy many design and manufacturing problems during the ensuing 60+ years. In parallel, root cause analysis techniques have helped in the investigation of spectacular failures, including the accident at the Three Mile Island Nuclear Power Plant and two space shuttle accidents. Fortunately—and for the betterment of the medical device industry, health providers, and patients alike—root cause analysis has been enthusiastically applied in the healthcare field for many problems, including adverse event analysis, customer complaint analysis of both single events and trending of multiple events, and CAPA (corrective and preventive action), as well as events related to product liability (Figure 0.1).

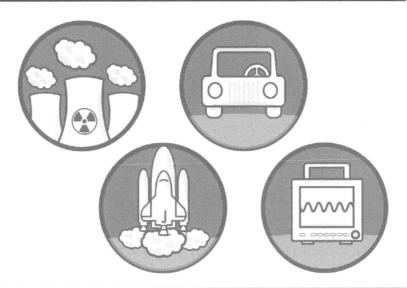

FIGURE 0.1 Clockwise from upper left: Symbols of a nuclear power plant, an automobile, a medical device, and a space shuttle. Official death toll resulting from accidents are: Three Mile Island = 0 (long-term health effects uncertain); space shuttle: 14 astronauts; car accidents in USA in 2014: 32,719; medical errors in USA in 2014: >200,000. (Adapted from James, J. T. 2013. A new, evidence-based estimate of patient harms associated with hospital care. *Journal of Patient Safety*, 9(3), 122–128.)

Let's talk more about this book now. I think you will find it to be well organized, taking you through a logical order of pertinent root cause analysis subject matter. The book educates readers on valuable topics such as the fundamentals of root cause analysis, the language of risk and root cause analysis, and regulatory expectations for the analysis of use errors. Additionally, several chapters provide practical instruction regarding identifying use errors, interviewing users about use errors, and user interface design flaws that might induce use errors.

Such design flaws are further exemplified through some very informative case studies in Chapter 12. These 30 examples graphically illustrate the issues that may be explored in a thorough analysis and the presentation style is very compelling. The examples cover a wide range of devices, including home-use products used by laypeople and highly complex devices used in clinical environments. I like the fact that each example concludes with suggestions on how to fix the problem that causes the use error. The simple illustrations are a great complement to the narrative explanations, in some cases clarifying design flaws that are difficult to appreciate just by reading words.

The examples are solid exemplars of the rigor with which the root cause analysis process should be applied. They show how root cause analysis leads from an understanding of the use error, its consequences, potential causes, and ultimately to mitigations and a range of solutions. In my view, these examples alone make the book a significant value.

The book also includes a discussion of the FDA mandates for application of best practice in human factors engineering. It is fairly well known that the FDA human factors product reviewers now require what is fundamentally a qualitative methodology for conducting usability tests, both formative and summative (validation). Unlike other regulated submissions to the FDA, such as clinical effectiveness, product stability, bioavailability, etc., human factors engineering is unique in not requiring inferential statistical evidence for medical device usability related to safety. This is because usability testing studies with proper statistical power would, to some manufacturers, be burdensome and impractical. Furthermore, the best way to understand the inevitable use errors that you are likely to observe in the final summative test is to do thorough root cause analysis. Then, designers must make the case that further redesign of the user interface is not practicable and that the remaining residual risk is acceptable because the clinical benefit of the device convincingly outweighs the residual risk. I know of no other way to justify the final design when you observe use errors in the summative test other than through root cause analysis. FDA guidance from both the Center for Devices and Radiological Health (CDRH) and Center for Drug Evaluation Research (CDER) reinforce the concept of risk/benefit trade-off.

To conclude this Foreword, I encourage readers to view root cause analysis as the sine qua non or the essence of good human factors. Industrial and user interface design is challenging, elusive, and a very creative part of usability engineering. However, due to limitations in the knowledge we have about human capabilities and limitations from the applied behavioral sciences, it is not easy to get early designs to be completely self-evident and intuitive. It takes hard work and a kind of brute force iterative process of design, testing, redesign, and retesting over multiple cycles to achieve a high-quality user interface. It would be almost impossible to learn from iterative cycles of design and testing without rigorous root cause analysis. This book makes a significant contribution to the literature on how to conduct root cause analysis as it applies to user interfaces.

Ed Israelski

Acknowledgments

We thank our colleagues at UL (Underwriters Laboratory)-Wiklund (a human factors engineering consulting firm) for their support. Our book cites many use errors related to those that occurred during usability tests conducted at UL-Wiklund. It also draws upon root cause analyses that we performed in close collaboration with our colleagues.

We particularly thank our professional family members Jonathan Kendler (our illustrator), Allison Strochlic, and Jon Tilliss, who energetically helped make Wiklund Research & Design a success, taking it to the point that it transitioned into the human factors engineering practice within UL.

We acknowledge other professionals who pioneered root cause analysis methods and wrote the papers and books cited in footnotes and listed in the book's list of resources. Our practical insights on root cause analysis stand on their original work.

Thanks go to Edmond Israelski, director of human factors at AbbVie, for writing the book's Foreword in which he shares his perspective on root cause analysis of medical device errors.

We thank our workmates Rachel Aronchick, Laura Birmingham, Stephanie Demarco Bartlett, Cory Costantino, Kelly Desharnais, Sami Durrani, Michael Geller, Limor Hochberg, Stephanie Larsen, and Frauke Schuurkamp-van Beek for their peer reviews of the book's draft content.

Merrick Kossack, manager of human factors engineering at Intuitive Surgical, Inc. (Sunnyvale, CA), was also generous to review our root cause analysis examples from a medical device developer's perspective and provided us with excellent advice.

Michael thanks his wife Amy for encouraging him to energetically pursue his interests, including writing about human factors engineering.

Finally, we collectively thank Taylor & Francis's Michael Slaughter for his enthusiastic response to our initial book proposal and steady support during its development and production, and Kathryn Everett for bringing the book swiftly from the manuscript stage to publication.

The authors thank the International Electrotechnical Commission (IEC) for permission to reproduce Information from its International Standards IEC 60601-1-6 ed.3.0 (2010) and IEC 62366-1 ed. 1.0 (2015). All such extracts are copyright of IEC, Geneva, Switzerland. All rights reserved. Further information on the IEC is available from www.iec.ch. IEC has no responsibility for the placement and context in which the extracts and contents are reproduced by the author, nor is IEC in any way responsible for the other content or accuracy therein.

Who Should Read This Book

Determining the root cause of use errors that people make when interacting with medical devices is key to design improvement and protecting people from harm. As such, this book's content should be of interest to a wide array of product development professionals and others who become involved in making healthcare delivery as safe and effective as possible, including the following:

✦ **Human factors specialists**—Individuals who are responsible for executing human factors engineering tasks, which include analyzing root causes of use errors detected during usability tests, clinical studies, and post-market surveillance.

✦ **Engineers and designers**—Individuals who might be asked to help perform human factors engineering work, as well as those who might participate in teams responsible for performing root cause analysis and responding to the findings by making changes to given devices. Such individuals might include mechanical, electrical, and systems engineers; project managers; software programmers; industrial designers; graphic designers; and people in many other associated professions.

✦ **Regulatory affairs specialists**—Individuals who manage their organizations' initiatives to comply with human factors standards that call for root cause analysis of use errors.

✦ **Quality assurance specialists**—Individuals who are concerned with meeting internal and externally applied quality standards for a variety of functions, including human factors engineering.

✦ **Risk managers and analysts**—Individuals who are responsible for their organizations' overall risk management efforts and who must incorporate root cause analysis results into their organizations' overall risk control schemes.

✦ **Patient safety specialists**—Individuals who seek to reduce the chance of harm to patients and the people who deliver care to them in clinical and non-clinical environments.

✦ **Regulators**—Individuals who (1) work for regulatory review and enforcement entities, such as the FDA, notified bodies in the European Union, and many more countries that evaluate risk mitigation efforts by manufacturers on behalf of federal entities, or (2) work for myriad organizations that advise the industry regarding regulatory strategy and responses to regulatory and legal enforcement actions (e.g., recalls, bans, consent decrees).

✦ **Students**—Individuals preparing to serve in the professional roles listed here.

Limitations of Our Advice

This book contains both factual information and content reflecting our professional judgment, complemented by hypothetical cases. Factual information includes definitions of the terms used to describe risk and root cause analysis, various regulatory requirements, and certain human factors engineering principles. Professional judgments include recommendations on how to approach root cause analysis, recognizing that capable professionals might take varying and equally productive approaches, and descriptions of user interface flaws that can induce use errors. Hypothetical cases of use errors and their root causes are sprinkled throughout many chapters and then concentrated in Chapter 12. Some of these cases were inspired by real cases, but we have changed the scenarios and eliminated product names to make the cases educational and to avoid targeting a particular medical device manufacturer.

This book references the most recent standards and guidance available at the time of publication. Readers should check for updates that might have bearing on how to conduct a root cause analysis to meet current standards and regulatory requirements and expectations.

To put our advice into proper context and identify other analytical options, we suggest that readers also consult other sources of guidance on root cause analysis as it is applied in the medical industry as well as in other industries (see Chapter 14 and the "Resources" section at the end of the book). Keep in mind that there is really no single way to perform root cause analysis and your needs might not be fully addressed by this book's contents.

Be aware that we have cited various root causes of the invented use errors, but that human factors engineering professionals could take issue with our conclusions. As such, our example root causes analyses should not be viewed as the definitive root cause of use errors that you might have to analyze in the future.

Naturally, we believe that we have converged on appropriate root causes, but as we state in Chapter 2, they remain no more than educated hypotheses in most cases. This is the true nature of most root cause analyses of use errors involving medical devices. The professional judgment that is usually inherent in a root cause analysis should not be viewed as a weakness, but rather as a fundamental and necessary characteristic given that we are dealing with human behavior and not machines. The practice of medicine is similar in this regard. Accurate diagnoses usually arise from both the consideration of factual knowledge and the application of judgment.

SIDEBAR 0.1   ROOT CAUSE ANALYSIS REQUIRES JUDGMENT IN THE SAME MANNER AS MEDICAL CARE

"The medical profession is 'a vocation in which a doctor's knowledge, clinical skills, and judgment are put in the service of protecting and restoring human well-being.' A basis of this profession is *clinical judgment*. It lies at the heart of the doctor's connoisseurship, expertise and skills, being 'almost as important as the technical ability to carry out the procedure itself.' Clinical judgment is developed through practice, experience, knowledge, and continuous critical analysis. It extends into all medical areas: diagnosis, therapy, communication, and decision making."[*]

---
[*] Kienle, G. and Kiene, H. 2011. "Clinical judgement [*sic*] and the medical profession." *Journal of Evaluation in Clinical Practice*, 17(4): 621–627. Available at http://www.ncbi.nlm.nih.gov/pmc/articles/PMC3170707/

SUMMARY DISCLAIMERS

This book was prepared by the authors in their personal capacities. The opinions expressed in it are the authors' own and do not reflect the view of their employer—UL LLC.

Any similarity to actual persons, living or dead, is purely coincidental.

Hypothetical cases and medical device examples reflect a broad base of professional experience. None are attributable to a single device. Product details have been described in generic ways.

The authors are not medical specialists. They applied a reasonable standard of care to describe sample harms associated with use errors. However, this information should not be used by others as a basis for determining such harms.

Authors

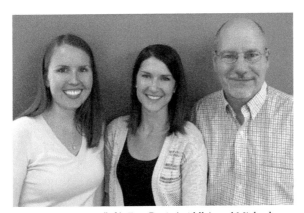

Andrea Dwyer (left), Erin Davis (middle), and Michael Wiklund (right).

Michael Wiklund serves as general manager of the human factors engineering (HFE) practice at UL-Wiklund. Before joining UL, he founded and managed his own HFE consulting firm—Wiklund Research & Design—which merged with UL in 2012. He has over 30 years of experience in human factors engineering, much of which has focused on medical technology development. His work has involved working with clients to optimize their products' safety, effectiveness, usability, and appeal. He is a certified human factors professional. His other publications (serving as author and/or editor) include *Usability Testing of Medical Devices, Handbook of*

Human Factors in Medical Device Design, Designing Usability into Medical Products, Medical Device and Equipment Design, and *Usability in Practice.* He is one of the primary contributors to today's most pertinent standards and guidelines on human factors engineering of medical devices: AAMI HE75 and IEC 62366. In addition to leading UL's human factors engineering practice, he serves as professor of the practice at Tufts University, where he teaches courses on HFE.

Andrea Dwyer serves as a managing human factors specialist at UL. In this role, she leads some of UL's most challenging user research and usability testing projects. She has authored numerous usability test reports that involve root cause analysis of use errors for medical devices ranging from insulin pumps to ultrasound systems to intraocular implants. Andrea also frequently composes usability engineering (i.e., HFE) program plans, administers usability tests, and develops HFE reports on behalf of UL's HFE clients.

Andrea earned her BS in human factors from Tufts University in 2010, where she received two prizes that honor achievement and excellence in human factors studies. To complement her studies, Andrea analyzed human factors issues associated with implanted devices, telemedicine, and assistive devices for senior citizens. In addition to her work in UL's HFE practice, she is currently a part-time graduate student in engineering management at Tufts University.

Erin Davis also serves as a managing human factors specialist at UL, working alongside her co-authors. She has several years' experience conducting human factors research in the field, including usability testing. Erin earned her MS in human factors engineering from Tufts University and her BS in biomedical engineering from Marquette University. To complement her undergraduate studies, Erin served as a systems engineering and human factors co-op at Baxter Healthcare and interned at the FDA. While earning her degrees, she conducted research on utility vehicle ergonomics, memory and fatigue, and completed her master's thesis on barriers and facilitators to orthopedic surgery. At UL-Wiklund, she develops and implements human factors engineering programs and leads projects requiring expertise in user research, design, and usability testing of medical devices.

Erin's other publications include "Cusp Catastrophe Models for Cognitive Workload and Fatigue in a Verbally-Cued Pictorial Memory Task" (*Human Factors*, 2012) and "Comparative Usability Study of Novel Auto-Injector and an Intranasal System for Naloxone Delivery" (*Pain and Therapy*, 2015). Erin won the best presentation award at the Human Factors and Ergonomics Society's 2013 New England Chapter Student Conference and is serving as the New England chapter's 2015 president.

1

Introduction

We have written *Medical Device Use Error: Root Cause Analysis* as a guide for human factors specialists and other professionals who are responsible for determining the causes of mistakes that people make when interacting with medical devices. We aspired to make the book a helpful complement to many other excellent books on the topic of root cause analysis (see the "Resources" section at the end of the book). We hope this book is particularly useful to readers in the field of human factors engineering (often referred to as HFE in shorthand) who work in the medical device industry.

Technology developers have been practicing root cause analysis for over 60 years, which is about as long as human factors engineering has been a recognized discipline; the Human Factors and Ergonomics Society was founded in 1957. The technique developed at a time when designers sought to improve the reliability (i.e., reduce the failure rate) of automobiles and more complex technologies, such as rockets. Most of you have probably seen the dramatic videos of early rockets exploding on the launch pad or during liftoff, and so you can understand the importance of identifying the root causes of such failures.

The root causes of failed rocket launches over many decades have included broken bolts, electrical failures, and O-ring erosion.[*] By comparison, the user interface-related root causes of harm resulting from medical device use errors have included flaws such as controls placed too close together, illegible information, and inaudible alarms. These examples tell us that even seemingly small flaws can lead to catastrophe.

Indeed, there have been plenty of injurious and fatal events linked to user interface design flaws that triggered use errors. Use errors have led to death due to such consequences as electric shock, radiation, drug overdoses and underdoses, infection, exsanguination (bleeding out), blunt trauma, and hypovolemia (severe dehydration). The deaths account for a small but significant percentage (perhaps 10%)[†] of all fatalities in the United States per year due to medical error that total in the range of 210,000–400,000 or more according to a recent estimate.[‡]

Let's now go back to the topic of conducting root cause analysis for the sake of identifying user interface design flaws and protecting medical device users from harm. Root cause analysis is a form of sleuthing. A systematic approach, complemented by creative insight, it offers the best chance of identifying the cause of a problem that could lead to harm. For example, analysts discovered that O-ring erosion led to hot gases escaping from one of the *Challenger* space shuttle's solid booster rockets, which in turn led to a catastrophic explosion. Analysts working in the medical industry determined that healthcare providers were inadvertently turning off an intravenous infusion pump rather than starting an essential infusion. In principle, once you know the root cause of a problem (prospectively or retrospectively), you can take corrective action, thereby reducing or eliminating the chance of the problem occurring in the future.

Fortunately for most of us who are healthcare consumers at various times, today's human factors engineering standards and regulations call for device developers who perform validation usability tests to conduct a root cause analysis of any use errors that occur during the test. The International Electrotechnical Commission's IEC 62366-1:2015[§] also suggests performing

---

[*] Blog: Metins Media & Math. "NASA's O-Ring Problem and the *Challenger* Disaster." Available at https://metinmediamath.wordpress.com/2013/12/03/nasas-o-ring-problem-and-the-challenger-disaster/

[†] Peter Carstensen, who led the FDA's human factors team until his retirement in 2008, suggested that 10% of fatal medical errors occurring annually in the United States at the time were due to use error. He made this suggestion at the Human Factors and Ergonomic Society's annual meeting in September 2008.

[‡] James, J. T. 2013. "A New, Evidence-Based Estimate of Patient Harms Associated with Hospital Care." *Journal of Patient Safety*, 9(3): 122–128.

[§] IEC 62366-1:2015, "Medical Devices—Part 1: Application of Usability Engineering to Medical Devices."

such analyses as a principal means to reduce the risk associated with use error. A similar standard of care applies to the investigation of adverse events involving medical devices.

Accordingly, there is an imperative for medical device manufacturers to analyze the root cause of use errors effectively. These analyses may lead to one of several possible conclusions regarding a particular use error that occurred during a usability test, including the following:

+ A user interface design flaw induced the use error.
+ The use error was purely due to human blunder.
+ The use error was triggered by a test method shortcoming (i.e., test artifact).

Bringing safe and effective medical devices to market hinges on a manufacturer's ability to recognize the true root causes of medical device use error and correct any identified user interface design flaws judged to pose an unacceptable risk. Similarly, a manufacturer's ability to bring commercially successful medical devices to market pivots on the quality of its root cause analysis, leading to insights on how to improve the device's usability, safety, and appeal.

Inadequate root cause analysis might lead to obstacles in the process of obtaining regulatory clearance for a new device, particularly if the analysis does not focus on design-related causes. Even if a device receives regulatory clearance, a faulty root cause analysis could open the opportunity for use errors to occur during actual medical care (as opposed to during usability test simulations), and possibly lead to user harm as well as significant consequences for the manufacturer.

Therefore, ensuring the safe and effective use of a medical device, as well as its commercial performance, rests in part on performing an effective root cause analysis of use errors. Most analyses will occur during product development, particularly following usability tests. But, such analyses also occur during adverse event investigation, as mentioned before. You will find that our book concentrates on the analysis that follows usability tests, but that the guidance usually applies well to adverse event postmortems.

Wrapping up this introduction, we hope this book helps you with the following:

+ Taking a systematic approach to identifying the root causes of use errors.
+ Understanding the regulatory imperatives to perform root cause analyses.

✦ Drawing upon feedback from device users, such as usability test participants and individuals involved in adverse events, to identify user interface design flaws that can lead to use errors.

✦ Drawing upon human factors engineering principles to identify user interface design flaws that induce use errors.

✦ Presenting root cause analysis results effectively in a usability test report.

✦ Determining possible user interface design mitigations to reduce the chance of use errors.

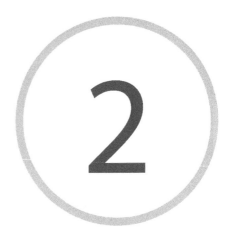

Our Root Cause Analysis Process

INTRODUCTION

As we stated in this book's introduction, we want to give readers helpful insights into how to perform root cause analysis of medical device use errors. Sometimes, the root cause of a use error seems obvious. Consider the case of a nurse who misread a parameter value displayed on a patient monitor as "63" instead of "68." You might jump to the conclusion that the numerals were too small given a reading distance of about 5 feet—that the 10 point (0.139 inch) high numerals were less than half the necessary height to read correctly from the given viewing distance based on human factors guidelines on making numerals legible (Figure 2.1).*

---

* At a viewing distance of 5 feet (60 inches), numerals would need to be a minimum of about 0.29 inches to subtend a minimum visual angle of 16 arc minutes (per ANSI/AAMI HE75:2009/(R)2013 guidance, see paragraph 19.4.1.2 Optimum character height, subparagraph a). Formula to calculate minimum character height: h = 2d tan(x/2), h = character height, d = viewing distance, and x = visual angle in radians. 1 radian equals 3437.747 arc minutes. Divide desired visual angle in arc minutes by 3437.747 to express visual angle in radians. Source: http://accessibility.gtri.gatech.edu/assistant/acc_info/font_size.php

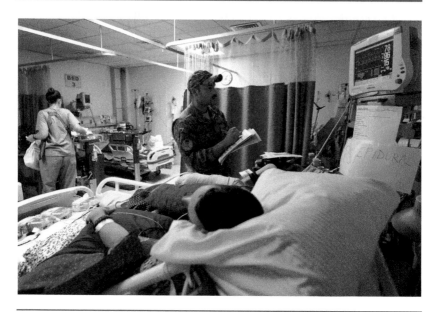

FIGURE 2.1   Nurse viewing patient monitor from greater than an arm's reach. (Note: The hypothetical number legibility problem discussed earlier is not specific to this monitor.) (From Air Force Medical Service. http://www.airforcemedicine.af.mil/)

Indeed, undersized numerals might be the dominant root cause of the cited use error. But, is it the only cause? Might there be additional root causes that acted in combination to induce the use error but are not as self-evident?

The answer is to expand the root cause analysis beyond "top of mind" causes (those identified by jumping to conclusions). In the preceding case, alternative, or at least contributing, root causes might include

+ Poor contrast between the numerals and background (e.g., black numbers on a medium-gray background).
+ Blur caused by vision impairment (e.g., cataract).
+ Glare on the screen.
+ Image vibration due to the monitor's use during transport (e.g., on a rolling stretcher, ambulance, or helicopter).

These legibility-compromising effects are shown in Figure 2.2, in this case, as they might manifest themselves on a handheld glucose meter.

So, what is a good approach to performing an expanded root cause analysis? The answer depends on many factors, including the use error characteristics and circumstances, how much effort you can and wish to invest in the analysis, the available time to perform an expanded analysis, and access to information that would support even deeper analysis.

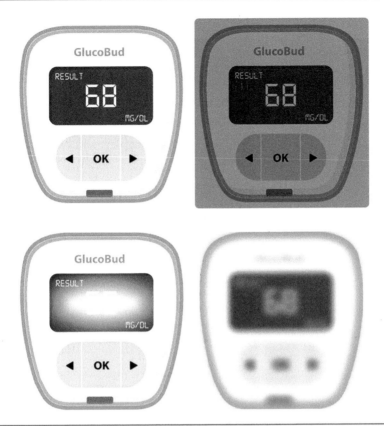

FIGURE 2.2   The measured glucose value at the upper left appears highly legible. Continuing clockwise, computer-generated effects show how reduced numeral-background contrast due to dim lighting, blur due to vision impairment, and glare could interfere with the measurement's legibility.

There are many documented approaches to conducting a root cause analysis (see Chapter 14 and the *Resources* section at the end of the book). That said, in the spirit of providing "one-stop shopping" for some readers, this chapter describes the root cause analysis workflow and strategy that we often employ. This process includes the following seven steps:

1. Define the use error
2. Identify provisional root causes
3. Analyze anecdotal evidence
4. Inspect device for user interface design flaws
5. Consider other contributing factors
6. Develop a final hypothesis
7. Report the results

STEP 1: DEFINE THE USE ERROR

Clearly define the use error (i.e., failure) of concern, including as much detail as possible. Document the sequence of events leading up to the failure and define the exact failure mode (e.g., did not start the infusion, entered the incorrect dose). To do this following a usability test, you should review all available data associated with the use error, including video recordings, notes from the test session, or the adverse event report. See Chapter 7 for guidance on detecting use errors during a usability test, clinical study, and post-market surveillance.

SIDEBAR 2.1 PROSPECTIVE VERSUS RETROSPECTIVE ROOT CAUSE ANALYSIS

In a prospective analysis, often employed early in a product's development, you speculate about what could happen in certain use scenarios. For example, you ask what use errors could occur when users operate a given medical device in dim lighting, while rushing through a task, after using a dissimilar device that performs the same basic function, etc. To support a prospective analysis, it can be helpful to complete a detailed task analysis* that examines all perceptual inputs, cognitive tasks, and actions associated with using a device to identify failure points.

After identifying each potential use error, you should perform root cause analyses to determine the foreseeable events that might lead to these failure points. You might end up with a long list of possibilities, but that is fine at this early stage of analysis. Also, there often are multiple contributing causes of a particular failure.

Retrospective root cause analysis is performed after an event occurs (e.g., you observed a use error during a usability test). When performing a retrospective analysis, you might have specific details on which to base your root cause analysis. For example, you might understand the exact sequence of events that led to a use error because you observed the event. Moreover, you might already have a general sense for why the error occurred, because you (or another

---

* FDA's "Draft Guidance for Industry and Food and Drug Administration Staff—Applying Human Factors and Usability Engineering to Optimize Medical Device Design" (issued June 22, 2011). Section 6.2.3, "Function and Task Analysis."

test administrator) already interviewed the usability test participant regarding the error's cause. Therefore, when performing retrospective root cause analysis, your focus is on the root causes that led to the specific instance of a use error, whereas with a prospective analysis you are anticipating possible root causes of errors that could occur in the future.

STEP 2: IDENTIFY PROVISIONAL ROOT CAUSES

Despite the aforementioned risk of jumping to conclusions, we think that identifying one or more provisional root causes is a good starting point as long as you are prepared to change your mind. You will likely have some sense of what caused a given mistake, so you might as well document it and then proceed to challenge your initial conclusion by performing additional analyses. For example, you might suspect that a usability test participant overlooked an important warning message because the warning is inconspicuous (e.g., placed on a device's back panel).

It can be helpful to have multiple analysts independently identify provisional root causes and then discuss their initial findings to converge on a set of provisional root causes. In other words, the analysts follow the same approach that human factors specialists take when they perform a heuristic analysis* of a user interface. The approach assumes that "two heads are better than one," and by extension, "three heads are better than two."

In fact, the Association for the Advancement of Medical Instruments' (AAMI's) technical information report on post-market surveillance suggests that there is value in having multiple individuals analyze use errors to determine root causes. The AAMI report goes further to suggest there is value in having several individuals participate in the process, particularly when analyzing a use error that occurred during actual device use in the field. Candidates who could support the analysis include the user who committed the use error, the user's manager or colleagues (if the use error occurred in a clinical setting), a biomedical engineer who is extensively familiar with the device under investigation, a device manufacturer representative (i.e., design

---

* Heuristic analysis of a user interface typically calls upon three human factors specialists to independently evaluate a design against heuristics (i.e., widely accepted design rules) and then convene to compare results and converge on a final set of findings.

engineer), the risk managers, and perhaps the clinical study safety officer (if the use error occurred in a clinical setting).*

STEP 3: ANALYZE ANECDOTAL EVIDENCE

Ideally, use error reports will state the potential causes of a given error that the person who made the mistake reported. Therefore, if you are administering a usability test during which a use error occurs, be sure to ask the participant to posit the cause (see Chapter 8). Asking participants the correct follow-up questions and collecting a sufficient amount of detail are necessary to enable a fruitful root cause analysis.

If you are investigating a use error that occurred during a device's actual use in the field (i.e., as part of a post-market surveillance effort), try to interview the person who committed the use error as soon as possible following the event. That said, conducting such an interview can pose challenges because the person or people involved might not always recollect past events accurately, openly, or honestly. You might be asking a healthcare professional to say something that seems self-incriminating, even if you approach the interview with a mindset to identify possible device flaws (not user flaws) that induced a use error. Therefore, the interviewee might not be forthcoming or even might be inaccessible because there is a pending lawsuit and she or he has been advised not to discuss the event in question.

If you have the opportunity to conduct an open and honest interview with a test participant or individual who experienced an error during actual device use, the user might be able to pinpoint a root cause or have no idea why she or he erred. As discussed in Chapter 9, users often blame themselves for mistakes as opposed to citing what a human factors specialist might consider to be the true root cause—a user interface design flaw. So, you must carefully consider participant-reported root causes, but recognize that participants' responses often only get you partway to the true root cause(s). Instead, you must rely on your professional experience and knowledge of human factors engineering principles when considering participant-reported root causes and determining if the most plausible root causes are actually design related.

In summary, you might learn a lot about a use error's root cause by talking to the person or people who made the mistake. But, beware of taking suggested root causes at face value. It's better to perform the other steps described in this root cause analysis process to complement what you learn during this step (Step 3).

---

* AAMI TIR50: 2014. Technical information report, "Post-market Surveillance of Use Error Management. Section 8.4, Evaluate Experience to Determine Root Cause," p. 22. Arlington, VA. 2014.

STEP 4: INSPECT DEVICE FOR USER INTERFACE DESIGN FLAWS

Perhaps the most fruitful step in root cause analysis is to inspect the given medical device for user interface design flaws. This step aligns well with the working assumption that most use errors are induced by design flaws and should not be attributed—at least not entirely—to user shortcomings (e.g., forgetfulness, inattention, fatigue). Human factors specialists are likely to possess a mental bank of user interface design heuristics and draw upon them to identify design flaws. In some sense, they will do this in Step 2 (identify provisional root causes). However, in lieu of perfect recall of applicable heuristics, specialists may also draw upon various reference sources (e.g., ANSI/AAMI HE75:2009/(R)2013) to check on best design practices and where a particular device deviates from them. See Chapter 10 for examples of common user interface design flaws that could have been avoided by considering heuristics. Additionally, many of the examples presented in Chapter 12 demonstrate the application of best practices to determine potential root causes of use error.

STEP 5: CONSIDER OTHER CONTRIBUTING FACTORS

In addition to identifying device-specific root causes, you should consider whether other factors contributed to the root cause, such as the following:

- Characteristics of the use environment, such as lighting, ambient noise level, precipitation, and distractions.
- User interface characteristics (or flaws) of other equipment in the environment.
- Test artifact, such as an unclear task prompt or insufficient realism due to a simulated use environment (e.g., a surgeon missing realistic tactile feedback when using a surgical tool to simulate a surgery).
- Participant's habits or experience with other devices that might influence the way she or he uses the test device (i.e., negative transfer).
- Participant's impairments, including physical (e.g., vision, hearing, dexterity) and cognitive (e.g., short-term memory loss).

SIDEBAR 2.2   CITING HABIT AND NEGATIVE TRANSFER AS ROOT CAUSES

You may attribute a use error to a participant's habit—an individual's behavior or customary practice as it relates to a given medical device's use. For example, it might be a participant's habit to discard a used needle in the household trash after injecting with his pen-injector at home. When participating in a usability test session and using a new pen-injector, the participant might take this same approach, discarding a used needle in the available trash can, rather than in the equally accessible sharps container.

A similar, but distinct, potential root cause is negative transfer. Negative transfer is when a user applies his or her knowledge of one product to another product, and consequently uses the other product incorrectly due to dissimilarities in operation between the two products. For example, a participant might remove only one of two adhesive patch liners from a transdermal patch because the patch she uses at home only has one liner. As such, the participant might not think to check for and remove a second liner when interacting with the new patch during the test session.

Although habit and negative transfer might be root causes that contribute to use error, in many cases one or more design-related root causes (i.e., user interface design flaws) are the primary contributors. In the transdermal patch example presented earlier, the participant did not remove the second liner in part due to negative transfer. However, the participant very likely overlooked the second liner because it was inconspicuous due to its transparent coloring and lack of a pull-tab. One more thing to keep in mind is that consequential actions due to habit and negative transfer might be avoidable if you account for these potentials and pursue design solutions that are not vulnerable to the problems.

STEP 6: DEVELOP A FINAL HYPOTHESIS

The next step in our root cause analysis process is to use the results of the preceding steps to develop a final hypothesis about what caused the given mistake. You would have likely identified several root causes in the course of performing Steps 1–5. To develop your final hypothesis, you challenge all of the candidate root causes and weed out those that inappropriately blame the user and those you ultimately consider to be the consequence of a deeper root cause. See the "five whys" section in Chapter 14 for a description of how asking "why" several times in a row can bring you to the true root cause. In the end, you may converge on one or more root causes.

We say hypothesis because the nature of the given use error and your analysis might not lead to a demonstrably true root cause or causes. There might always be a degree of speculation, recognizing that human behavior is variable and difficult to characterize fully. The point of performing a systematic root cause analysis is to minimize the level of speculation, bringing to bear evidence and sometimes a strong dose of professional judgment to arrive at the best possible explanation for a use error that might otherwise defy absolute attribution. This sets the stage for risk mitigation—putting in place protections against future use errors.

STEP 7: REPORT THE RESULTS

The final step is to report the root cause analysis results. In Step 7, you will have arrived at a strong hypothesis regarding a use error's cause or causes. Your report should cite the evidence leading to the hypothesis. Reports may be terse or expansive depending on their purpose and intended audience (e.g., design team members, regulators). In Chapter 11, we describe the content that we normally include in such reports and provide a few example reports.

NEXT STEPS

After completing a root cause analysis, the next task is to perform a residual risk analysis to determine whether the risk associated with the use error warrants further mitigation. For more details on residual risk analysis, see Chapter 11.

In the course of completing your residual risk analysis, you might determine that the risk is unacceptably high and that it is necessary to mitigate the risk to reduce the likelihood of future failures. If you identified the root cause(s) by (1) analyzing a use error that occurred during usability testing or (2) predicting the use error based on prospective analysis, your task is to modify the device in development so as to eliminate or further mitigate the risk. If the use error occurred during use with an existing (i.e., commercially available) medical device, then your task is to identify the appropriate corrective action to prevent or mitigate the consequences of future use errors involving the device. The latter option would likely be part of a so-called CAPA (standing for corrective and preventive action). The corrective action you identify might be to change the device user interface, in which case Chapter 13 should be a helpful resource.

SIDEBAR 2.3   WHAT IS A CAPA?

CAPA stands for corrective and preventive action. In the medical industry, CAPA is a quality assurance mechanism that is closely tied to good manufacturing practices (GMP) and is prescribed by multiple international standards as a response to known deviations from quality goals and to adverse events. A CAPA program calls for manufacturers to identify and investigate device quality problems, including harms that occurred as a consequence of actual device use (as opposed to simulated use), and to take appropriate and effective corrective and/or preventive action to prevent a recurrence. Verifying or validating corrective and preventive actions, communicating corrective and preventive action activities to responsible people, providing relevant information for management review, and documenting these activities are essential steps toward effectively addressing quality problems, preventing their recurrence, and preventing or minimizing device failures.[*]

---

[*] "Inspections, Compliance, Enforcement, and Criminal Investigations, Corrective and Preventive Actions (CAPA)." Available at http://www.fda.gov/iceci/inspections/inspectionguides/ucm170612.htm

---

SIDEBAR 2.4   PERFORM ADDITIONAL TYPES OF ROOT CAUSE ANALYSES

In Chapter 14, we review several root cause analysis techniques that you may choose to use to analyze a use error in different ways. Such techniques as the five whys, Ishikawa diagramming, drawing AcciMaps, and others can place a use error in a broader context that looks beyond user interface design flaws and considers aspects of the use environment and culture, for example.

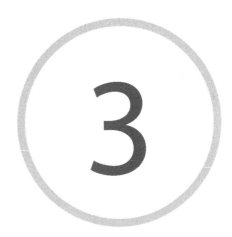

The Regulatory Imperative to Perform Root Cause Analysis

There is a definitive, regulator-driven need to perform root cause analysis of use errors detected in a summative (i.e., validation) usability test of a medical device. In some cases, there is also a need to perform such analyses of adverse events. Root cause analysis is a bridge between detecting use errors and determining ways to prevent them.

FDA REGULATIONS

On October 7, 1996, FDA modified the Quality System Regulation* (QSR) in a manner that ostensibly called upon medical device manufacturers to apply human factors engineering to devices that are subject to design con-

---

* CFR—Code of Federal Regulations, Title 21, "Food and Drugs," Chapter I, "Food and Drug Administration," Department of Health and Human Services, Subchapter H, "Medical Devices," Part 820, "Quality System Regulation." Available at http://www.accessdata.fda.gov/scripts/cdrh/cfdocs/cfcfr/CFRSearch.cfm?CFRPart=820&showFR=1

trols (e.g., a few Class I devices and all Class II and III devices). The change was finalized and went into effect one year later. The pertinent QSR text follows:

(c) *Design input.* Each manufacturer shall establish and maintain procedures to ensure that the design requirements relating to a device are appropriate and address the intended use of the device, including the needs of the user and patient. The procedures shall include a mechanism for addressing incomplete, ambiguous, or conflicting requirements. The design input requirements shall be documented and shall be reviewed and approved by a designated individual(s). The approval, including the date and signature of the individual(s) approving the requirements, shall be documented.

(f) *Design verification.* Each manufacturer shall establish and maintain procedures for verifying the device design. Design verification shall confirm that the design output meets the design input requirements. The results of the design verification, including identification of the design, method(s), the date, and the individual(s) performing the verification, shall be documented in the DHF.

(g) *Design validation.* Each manufacturer shall establish and maintain procedures for validating the device design. Design validation shall be performed under defined operating conditions on initial production units, lots, or batches, or their equivalents. Design validation shall ensure that devices conform to defined user needs and intended uses and shall include testing of production units under actual or simulated use conditions. Design validation shall include software validation and risk analysis, where appropriate. The results of the design validation, including identification of the design, method(s), the date, and the individual(s) performing the validation, shall be documented in the DHF.

The call to action is subtle in the sense that the term "human factors engineering" and one of the key techniques—usability testing—are not mentioned specifically. However, the updated QSR empowered the FDA to examine the human factors suitability of medical device submissions (e.g., Pre-IDE, IDE, 510(k), PMA).* The statement "testing of production units under actual or simulated use conditions" in paragraph (g) is essentially a call for usability testing.

After years of what some people judged to be low-key enforcement, the FDA seemed to step up its enforcement in the mid-2000s. Reportedly, the wide range in quality of human factors engineering data in medical device submissions led FDA to publish a guide on the subject in 2011. Though the guide was termed a draft and not ready for implementation per se, it nonetheless described the approach FDA had and would continue to take when reviewing human factors engineering data. So, in the key sense, there was nothing "draft" about the guidance except that it was subject to change. FDA received extensive comments on the draft document and reportedly will issue final guidance in the near future, perhaps before this book is published. As such, readers should review the most up-to-date human factors engineering guidance from FDA.

FDA's HFE guidance† (Section 10.1.5, "Interpretation of Validation Test Results and Addressing Problems") states:

> Problems with the design of the device, labeling, or training requirements should have been identified and addressed prior to validation testing. When use problems do occur during validation testing, this usually indicates that the previous HFE/UE steps were not performed adequately. **The root causes of problems identified during validation testing should be evaluated from the perspective of the test participants involved and direct performance data will support this determination.** Data analysis should include subjective feedback regarding critical task experience, difficulties, "close calls," and any task failures by test participants. Depending on the extent of the risk mitigation strategies required, revalidation may be necessary. You should address failures and difficulties associated with greater than minimal risk and attributable to the user interface by designing and implementing risk mitigation strategies and retesting those elements to confirm their success at reducing risks to acceptable levels without introducing any new risks.

---

* Applicability as described by the FDA on its webpage titled "Human Factors and Medical Devices," Human Factors Program at FDA, Human Factors at Center for Devices and Radiological Health (CDRH), Office of Device Evaluation (ODE). Available at http://www.accessdata.fda.gov/scripts/cdrh/cfdocs/cfcfr/CFRSearch.cfm?CFRPart=820&showFR=1&subpartNode=21:8.0.1.1.12.3

† FDA's "Draft Guidance for Industry and Food and Drug Administration Staff—Applying Human Factors and Usability Engineering to Optimize Medical Device Design" (issued June 22, 2011).

In this guidance, FDA calls upon manufacturers to perform root cause analysis of use errors that occur during a summative usability test. In the course of performing such root cause analysis, you should consider both a participant's perspective on the use error that occurred and task performance data (e.g., the test personnel's observations) collected during the test session.

EUROPEAN UNION REGULATIONS

The European Union (EU) issues directives (i.e., legislative acts) that apply to the member states. As of early 2015, the 28 states included Austria, Belgium, Bulgaria, Croatia, Republic of Cyprus, Czech Republic, Denmark, Estonia, Finland, France, Germany, Greece, Hungary, Ireland, Italy, Latvia, Lithuania, Luxembourg, Malta, Netherlands, Poland, Portugal, Romania, Slovakia, Slovenia, Spain, Sweden, and the United Kingdom.[*]

In "Medical Device Directive 93/42/EEC," the EU expects medical device manufacturers to comply with the essential requirements, and indirectly the European (EN) version of 60601, third edition, including collateral (i.e., horizontal) standard IEC 62366-1:2015.[†] As of June 1, 2012. IEC 60601, second edition, did not require a manufacturer to comply with the usability standard to declare conformance with the overarching standard and CE mark a Class IIa, IIb, or III medical devices.[‡]

IEC 62366-1:2015 directly addresses the topic of root cause analysis. It states:

> The data from the summative evaluation shall be analyzed to identify the potential consequences of all use errors that occurred. If the consequences can be linked to a hazardous situation, the root cause of each use error shall be determined. The root causes should be determined based on observations of user performance and subjective comments from the user related to that performance.

---

[*] List of European Union member states available at http://en.wikipedia.org/wiki/Member_state_of_the_European_Union#List

[†] IEC 62366-1:2015, "Medical Devices—Part 1: Application of Usability Engineering to Medical Devices."

[‡] "Medical Devices: Guidance Document, Classification of Medical Devices," MEDDEV 2. 4/1 Rev. June 9, 2010. Available at http://ec.europa.eu/health/medical-devices/files/meddev/2_4_1_rev_9_classification_en.pdf

OTHER REGULATORS

Regulators with authority in countries other than the United States and EU member states expect manufacturers to uphold IEC 60601 and, therefore, meet the requirements set forth in the original or most up-to-date version of IEC 62366. Such countries include Canada, Japan, Singapore, South Korea, and Taiwan. Given the specific and limited focus of this book, we advise readers to consult regulatory affairs specialists for more details about human factors engineering requirements in these regions.

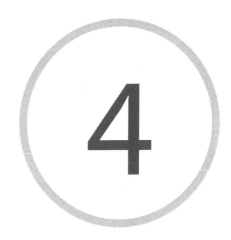

Applicable Standards
and Guidelines

The following standards and guidelines pertain to the root cause analysis of medical device use errors and helped shape the guidance provided in this book.

1. *U.S. Food and Drug Administration (Silver Spring, Maryland):* "Draft Guidance for Industry and Food and Drug Administration Staff— Applying Human Factors and Usability Engineering to Optimize Medical Device Design" (issued June 22, 2011).

SCOPE*

[FDA's] guidance provides recommendations for medical device design optimization through human factors analysis, testing, and validation. The intent is to improve the quality of the device user interface such

---

* Available at http://www.fda.gov/MedicalDevices/DeviceRegulationandGuidance/ GuidanceDocuments/ucm259748.htm

that errors that occur during use of the device are either eliminated or reduced. The recommendations in this document apply whenever a manufacturer performs human factors testing for a device.

As part of their design controls* manufacturers conduct a risk analysis that includes risks associated with device use. If the results of this analysis indicate that there is a moderate to high risk of use error, or if a manufacturer is modifying a marketed device due to problems associated with use, particularly as a corrective and preventive action (CAPA), then the manufacturer should perform appropriate human factors testing according to this guidance document. Additionally, FDA staff may request human factors testing if (i) submission of human factors information is required (for example, as a special control); (ii) submission of human factors information is recommended in a specific guidance for a device type and the manufacturer cannot justify forgoing such testing; or (iii) on a for-cause basis if it is the least burdensome method to address FDA's concerns regarding human factors issues. Under these circumstances, manufacturers should provide FDA with a report that summarizes the human factors processes, evaluations, and results of validation testing as part of their premarket applications or submissions (see Appendix A).†

---

* 21 CFR 820.30.

† Appendix A HFE/UE report. Available at http://www.fda.gov/MedicalDevices/DeviceRegulationandGuidance/GuidanceDocuments/ucm259748.htm#a

As indicated in the preceding excerpt, FDA's guidance describes the human factors engineering activities the agency expects manufacturers to perform when developing medical devices. Importantly, the agency expects manufacturers to conduct a summative (i.e., validation) usability test to document all safety-related use errors (as well as close calls and difficulties), and then to perform root cause analyses of these events. The root cause analyses should focus more on the device's user interface shortcomings (i.e., flaws) and less on user fallibilities.

During conference presentations and in letters to individual manufacturers, FDA representatives have made comments that suggest the agency is not concerned with use errors that are strictly usability related and have no bearing on personal safety or the ability of users to perform essential tasks. As such, manufacturers may choose to perform a root cause analysis of non-safety-related use errors at their own discretion. If a manufacturer chooses to diagnose the cause of all user interaction problems, it is likely to be in the pursuit of design excellence and not simply to satisfy FDA's or any other regulator's expectations.

2. *International Standards Organization (Geneva, Switzerland):* ISO 13485:2003 "Medical Devices—Quality Management Systems— Requirements for Regulatory Purposes."

ABSTRACT*

ISO 13485:2003 specifies requirements for a quality management system where an organization needs to demonstrate its ability to provide medical devices and related services that consistently meet customer requirements and regulatory requirements applicable to medical devices and related services.

The primary objective of ISO 13485:2003 is to facilitate harmonized medical device regulatory requirements for quality management systems. As a result, it includes some particular requirements for medical devices and excludes some of the requirements of ISO 9001 that are not appropriate as regulatory requirements. Because of these exclusions, organizations whose quality management systems conform to this International Standard cannot claim conformity to ISO 9001 unless their quality management systems conform to all the requirements of ISO 9001.

All requirements of ISO 13485:2003 are specific to organizations providing medical devices, regardless of the type or size of the organization.

If regulatory requirements permit exclusions of design and development controls, this can be used as a justification for their exclusion from the quality management system. These regulations can provide alternative arrangements that are to be addressed in the quality management system. It is the responsibility of the organization to ensure that claims of conformity with ISO 13485:2003 reflect exclusion of design and development controls.

If any requirement(s) in Clause 7 of ISO 13485:2003 is(are) not applicable due to the nature of the medical device(s) for which the quality management system is applied, the organization does not need to include such a requirement(s) in its quality management system.

The processes required by ISO 13485:2003, which are applicable to the medical device(s), but which are not performed by the organization, are the responsibility of the organization and are accounted for in the organization's quality management system.

---

* Available at http://www.iso.org/iso/catalogue_detail?csnumber=36786

ISO 13485:2003 calls upon medical device manufacturers to establish a quality management system. In doing so, the standard implicitly requires manufacturers to implement a risk management process, which in turn calls for the assessment and reduction of use-related risks. Recognizing that performing root cause analyses is a way to identify opportunities to lower risks, one could say that performing such analyses is also implicit.

3. *International Standard Organization (Geneva, Switzerland):* ISO 14971:2007 "Medical Devices—Application of Risk Management to Medical Devices"

ABSTRACT*

ISO 14971:2007 specifies a process for a manufacturer to identify the hazards associated with medical devices, including in vitro diagnostic (IVD) medical devices, to estimate and evaluate the associated risks, to control these risks, and to monitor the effectiveness of the controls.

The requirements of ISO 14971:2007 are applicable to all stages of the life cycle of a medical device.

---

* Available at http://www.iso.org/iso/catalogue_detail?csnumber=38193

By calling upon manufacturers to identify risks associated with the use of medical devices, ISO 14971:2007 establishes the expectation that manufacturers will treat use errors as one of many kinds of failures—akin to the risk associated with an electrical short circuit—that pose a risk. The document provides guidance on how to estimate the level of risk by considering the likelihood of a failure occurring and the severity of the potential harm that might result. Such estimates can be completed using a variety of techniques, but most are performed within the framework of a failure modes and effects analysis (FMEA) that leads to a table of potential failure modes and their associated risks before and after the application of risk control measures (i.e., remedies). As such, a manufacturer will devote a portion of an FMEA table (or the output of another risk estimation technique) to use errors, just as it will devote a portion to electrical failures such as the one just described.

4. *International Electrotechnical Commission (Geneva, Switzerland):* IEC 60601-1-6 "Medical electrical equipment—Part 1–6: General Requirements for Basic Safety and Essential Performance—Collateral Standard: Usability"

ABSTRACT*

IEC 60601-1-6:2010 specifies a process for a manufacturer to analyse, specify, design, verify, and validate usability, as it relates to basic safety and essential performance of medical electrical equipment. This usability engineering process assesses and mitigates risks caused by usability problems associated with correct use and use errors, i.e., normal use. It can be used to identify but does not assess or mitigate risks associated with abnormal use. If the usability engineering process detailed in this collateral standard has been complied with and the acceptance criteria documented in the usability validation plan have been met (see 5.9 of IEC 62366:2007), then the residual risks, as defined in ISO 14971, associated with usability of [medical electrical] equipment are presumed to be acceptable, unless there is objective evidence to the contrary (see 4.1.2 of IEC 62366:2007). The object of this collateral standard is to specify general requirements that are in addition to those of the general standard and to serve as the basis for particular standards. This document cancels and replaces the second edition of IEC 60601-1-6 which has been technically revised. It was revised to align with the usability engineering process in IEC 62366. To allow for equipment manufacturers and testing organizations to make products and to equip themselves for conducting revised tests in accordance with this third edition, it is recommended by SC 62A that the content of this document not be adopted for mandatory implementation earlier than 3 years from the date of publication for equipment newly designed and not earlier than 5 years from the date of publication for equipment already in production.

---

* Available at https://webstore.iec.ch/publication/2596

IEC 60601-1-6 is essentially the predecessor to IEC 62366:2007, which, in turn, is the predecessor to IEC 62366-1:2015. IEC first released IEC 60601-1-6 in 2004. Subsequently, IEC determined that the collateral standard should be extended to cover a wider range of medical devices rather than just electromechanical devices. Therefore, in 2007, it released what is essentially an updated version of the original standard, now naming it IEC 62366. See the following discussion of IEC 62366-1:2015 for more details.

5. *International Electrotechnical Commission (Geneva, Switzerland):*
    IEC 62366-1:2015 "Medical Devices—Part 1: Application of Usability
    Engineering to Medical Devices"

ABSTRACT*

[IEC 62366-1:2015] specifies a process for a manufacturer to analyse,
specify, develop, and evaluate the usability of a medical device as it relates
to safety. This usability engineering (human factors engineering) process
permits the manufacturer to assess and mitigate risks associated with
correct use and use errors, i.e., normal use. It can be used to identify but
does not assess or mitigate risks associated with abnormal use. This first
edition of IEC 62366-1, together with the first edition of IEC 62366-2
(not published yet), cancels and replaces the first edition of IEC 62366
published in 2007 and its Amendment 1:2014. Part 1 has been updated
to include contemporary concepts of usability engineering, while also
streamlining the process. It strengthens links to ISO 14971:2007 and the
related methods of risk management as applied to safety related aspects
of medical device user interfaces. Part 2, once published, will contain
tutorial information to assist manufactures in complying with Part 1, as
well as offering more detailed descriptions of usability engineering methods that can be applied more generally to medical devices that go beyond
safety-related aspects of medical device user interfaces.

---

* Available at https://webstore.iec.ch/publication/21863

IEC 62366-1:2015 parallels FDA's guidance (see the "Scope" box
at the beginning of this chapter), calling upon manufacturers to
conduct a summative (i.e., validation) usability test, to document all
safety-related use errors (as well as close calls and difficulties), and
then to perform a root cause analysis of these events.

Note: In 2014, IEC released Amendment 1 (Annex K) to IEC
62366:2007 to address the usability engineering (aka human factors
engineering) requirements that pertain to so-called legacy devices:
devices that were originally brought to market prior to when IEC
published its usability engineering requirements. The amendment
called for a retrospective assessment of use-related risk to determine if further risk control measures are warranted. The original
amendment's content now takes the form of "Annex C—Evaluation
of a User Interface of Unknown Provenance (UOUP)" in the updated
standard.

SUMMARY

Taken as a whole, the standards and guidance described in this chapter call upon manufacturers to take the following steps:

1. **Quality system.** Establish a quality system that includes a risk management process. This process must consider a wide range of risks including those related to users' interactions with medical devices.

2. **Validation usability test.** Conduct a validation (i.e., summative) usability test to determine if users are able to perform higher risk tasks with a given medical device in a safe and effective manner. The presumption is that the risk associated with performing the selected tasks has been reduced by means of various risk control measures, so the validation test seeks to prove that the measures worked.

3. **Root cause analysis.** Determine the root cause(s) of any user interaction problems (e.g., safety-related use errors, close calls, and difficulties) that occur during a validation usability test as an input to a residual risk analysis.

4. **Residual risk analysis.** Perform a residual risk analysis of safety-related user interaction problems to determine if there is a need and means to reduce the cited risks.

5. **Additional risk control measures.** Implement the necessary and feasible further risk control measures and, if necessary, conduct a follow-up validation usability test.

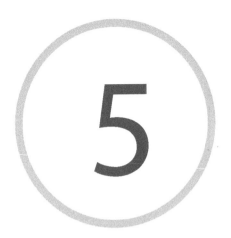

The Language of Risk and Root Cause Analysis

INTRODUCTION

Risk analysis calls for the use of precise language, dismissing vernacular and connotation in favor of defined terms. It is a smart approach that helps prevent miscommunication. Given that a thorough understanding of risk analysis is helpful when performing root cause analysis of use errors, newcomers would be well served to learn the language and avoid using risk and root cause analysis terms imprecisely.

As you may already know or come to understand by learning the terms defined in this chapter, it is accurate to say that a metal box's sharp edge is a hazard that can cause harm and, therefore, poses a risk. However, it is technically inaccurate to say that a sharp edge is a risk. As discussed later, the term "risk" is multivariate, accounting for both the likelihood of harm occurring and the severity of the harm.

Here are the ISO 14971:2007* definitions (in italics) and some clarifications for key terms.

Risk analysis—Systematic use of available information to identify hazards, to define harms, and to estimate the risk.

Medical companies normally establish detailed standard operating procedures (SOPs) describing their approach to risk analysis. ISO 14971:2007 provides detailed guidance on the topic.

Harm—Physical injury or damage to the health of people, or damage to property or the environment.

Potential harms include the following:

+ Heart fibrillation
+ Infection
+ Air embolism
+ Drug overdose
+ Delay in therapy
+ Burn
+ Crushed finger

Hazard—Potential source of harm.
Sample hazards include the following:

+ *Biological hazards* such as bacteria, viruses, and non-sterile material.
+ *Chemical hazards* such as high drug concentration, incorrect drug, or expired drug.
+ *Energy hazards* such as radiation, electricity, high temperature, or vibration.
+ *Operational hazards* such as an incorrect measurement, incorrectly assembled device, or incorrect flow rate.
+ *Physical hazards* such as a pinch point, an exposed needle, or repetitive movements.

Hazardous situation—Circumstance in which people, property, or the environment are exposed to one or more hazard(s).

Example hazardous situations include the following:

+ *Noisy emergency department.* A nurse is working in a hospital's emergency department in which there is considerable noise produced by people speaking loudly, equipment movement, room heating/cooling fans, telephones ringing, and frequent and concurrent equipment

---

* ISO 14971:2007. "Medical Devices—Application of Risk Management to Medical Devices."

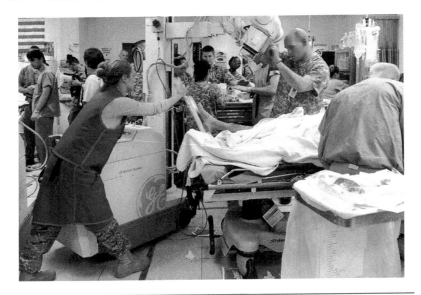

FIGURE 5.1   Emergency departments can have high ambient noise levels due to multiple conversations, equipment noise, overhead pages, and ringing phones. (From U.S. Department of Defense. U.S. Air Force photo by Tech. Sgt. Jeromy K. Cross. Accessed from http://www.defense.gov/dodcmsshare/photoessay/2010-02/hires_100209-F-0571C-331a.jpg)

alarms. As a result, a nurse does not detect a particular patient monitor's apnea (i.e., patient not breathing) alarm and the patient suffers a lack of oxygen (Figure 5.1).

✦ *Incomplete dose remaining in pen-injector.* A layperson who treats his diabetes with insulin injections requires 20 units of insulin in the morning before eating breakfast. The insulin pen-injector that he has been using for several days has only 8 units of insulin remaining in it. He must split his total dose between two insulin pen-injectors. As a result, the layperson commits a math error and delivers too much insulin (i.e., overdoses).

✦ *Occluded chest drain.* A patient who has a chest drain is undergoing a lengthy surgery. The chest drain becomes occluded (i.e., blocked). Nearby, there is a machine intended to provide high suction at the surgical site for the purpose of removing blood and other kinds of waste. As a result, a member of the surgical team attaches the high suction line to the chest tube to remove the occlusion, thereby applying a high vacuum to the patient's lung and causing tissue damage.

Note: Additional examples are provided in IEC 62366-1:2015, "Annex B—Examples of Possible Hazardous Situations Related to Usability" (Figure 5.2).

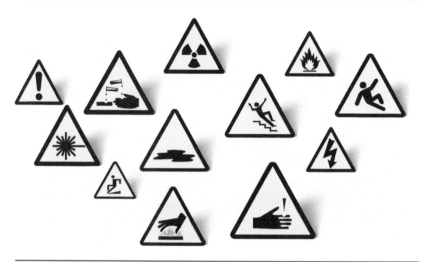

FIGURE 5.2   Sample caution signs for various hazardous situations.

Intended use—Intended purpose for which a product, process, or service is intended according to the specifications, instructions, and information provided by the manufacturer.

Examples of intended use include the following:

✦ *Insulin pump.* This device, which can be programmed to deliver a continuous stream of insulin, might be intended for use by teenagers and adults who have diabetes, but not by a young (e.g., <13 years of age), unsupervised child.

✦ *Surgical robot.* This device, which enables surgeons to perform precise surgeries via remote manipulators, might be intended for use only by qualified surgeons who have received intensive, week-long training regarding the device's use.

✦ *Nebulizer.* This device, which turns fluid medicine (e.g., Dornase Alfa to treat cystic fibrosis) into an aerosol for inhalation, might be suitable for the delivery of certain drugs but not others.

Use error—Act or omission of an act that results in a different medical device response than that intended by the manufacturer or expected by the user.

The term "use error" is generally synonymous with the term "mistake," although some specialists use the term "mistake" technically only to describe cases when someone acts intentionally but incorrectly (see Chapter 6). In the context of a use error, a person has done the wrong thing (an act of omission or commission) regardless of whether the device or circumstances of use induced the error.

Sample use errors include the following:

+ *Programs wrong fluid delivery rate.* A nurse programs an infu-sion pump to deliver a fluid at a rate of 100 mL/hour when the prescription said 10 mL/hour. This use error (of commission) leads to a drug overdose.
+ *Does not agitate drug.* A user of a multi-use auto-injector does not agitate a two-part drug contained within the device that is prone to separation between device uses. This use error (of omission) leads to an injection of the wrong proportions of the drug components.
+ *Does not open clamp.* A dialysis technician neglects to open a clamp on a bag of dialysate. This use error (of omission) prevents the proper flow of dialysate through a dialysis machine's tubing set and into the patient's body.

Likelihood—Estimate of the frequency of a harmful event.

Likelihood (aka frequency) is usually defined using a scale. The follow-ing is a common scale with five levels*:

Term	Examples of Probability Range
Frequent	≥1 in 1000
Probable	<1 in 1,000 and ≥1 in 10,000
Occasional	<1 in 10,000 and ≥1 in 100,000
Remote	<1 in 100,000 and ≥1 in 1,000,000
Improbable	<1 in 1,000,000

The following are a few sample use errors and the associated likelihood ratings (i.e., the likelihood the use error will occur and result in harm):

Likelihood Rating	Term	Example Use Error
5	Frequent	Patient does not log dose using dose adherence smartphone application
4	Probable	Patient drops device
3	Occasional	Patient does not detect audible alarm
2	Remote	Patient does not install battery
1	Improbable	Patient uses device with wrong power cord

---

* ISO 14971:2007. "Medical devices—Application of Risk Management to Medical Devices," Section D.3.4.2, "Semi-quantitative Analysis," Table D.4.

Severity—Measure of the possible consequences of a hazard.

As mentioned before, the severity of a harm is usually defined using a scale. The following is a common scale with five levels[*]:

Term	Possible Description
Catastrophic	Results in patient death
Critical	Results in permanent impairment or life-threatening injury
Serious	Results in injury or impairment requiring professional medical intervention
Minor	Results in temporary injury or impairment not requiring professional medical intervention
Negligible	Inconvenience or temporary discomfort

These levels can be further defined in terms of the permanence of the harm.

The following are a few sample harms and their associated severity ratings:

Severity Rating	Term	Example Harm
5	Catastrophic	Air embolism
4	Critical	Systemic infection
3	Serious	Allergic reaction
2	Minor	Delayed therapy
1	Negligible	Injection site discomfort

The process of assigning likelihood and severity values to use errors and harms, respectively, is called risk estimation.

Risk—Combination of the probability of occurrence of harm and the severity of that harm.

Typically, risk is quantified by multiplying a numerical rating of likelihood (e.g., 3 = occasional, on a scale of 1 = improbable and 5 = frequent) by a numerical rating of the severity of the potential harm (e.g., 3 = serious, on a scale of 1 = negligible and 5 = catastrophic) resulting in a so-called risk priority number (RPN) of $3 \times 3 = 9$ (Figure 5.3). As such, risk is not synonymous with the chance of a harm occurring, even though the term is often used to convey this meaning by nonspecialists.

Accordingly, there is high risk when the likelihood and severity of harm are both high. Conversely, there is low risk when the likelihood and severity of harm are both low. What about high–low combinations? A risk might

---

[*] ISO 14971:2007. "Medical Devices—Application of Risk Management to Medical Devices," Section D.3.4.2, "Semi-quantitative Analysis," Table D.3.

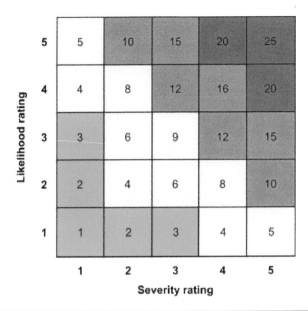

FIGURE 5.3   Graphical depiction of risk levels that uses color to indicate risks that are in a more acceptable versus less acceptable range.

very well be unacceptable if the likelihood is low but the potential severity of the harm is high.

Note that there are other ways to calculate risk. For example, one approach factors in the chance that a user will detect an error (i.e., the detectability) and, presumably, correct it before significant harm can occur.

Risk evaluation—Process of comparing the estimated risk against given risk criteria to determine the acceptability of the risk.

Analysts evaluating the risk posed by a medical device usually look to ISO 14971:2007 for guidance on what constitutes acceptable risk, often establishing a numerical limit for which risks warrant risk control measures and which ones do not. For example, a manufacturer might consider risks of RPN 8 or higher to be unacceptable, and therefore warrant risk mitigation.

When evaluating risks, three outcomes are possible:

✦ The risk is too high and therefore unacceptable.
✦ The risk is very low (i.e., negligible) and therefore acceptable.
✦ The risk is neither negligible nor so high as to be considered unacceptable.

In the last case, ISO 14971:2007 recommends that manufacturers reduce the risk such that the risk is "as low as reasonably practicable" or ALARP.

This approach weighs the benefits for further risk reduction against the cost of implementing additional risk control measures. As a result, a manufacturer might deem a risk acceptable if the manufacturer considers the cost of further reducing the risk too high.

SIDEBAR 5.1   ALARP VERSUS ALAP

ISO 14971:2007 requires manufacturers to determine, for each identified hazardous situation, whether risk reduction is required by applying the risk criteria identified in the risk management plan. ISO 14971:2007 also indicates that risks be driven as low as reasonably practicable. However, the European Union (EU) version of the standard (EN ISO 14971:2012) calls upon manufacturers to follow a somewhat different risk acceptability approach. Specifically, the EU version includes a deviation from the baseline standard, stating that manufacturers must reduce risks to "as low as possible" (ALAP), rather than "as low as reasonably practicable" (ALARP).

When following the ALARP approach, manufacturers should reduce unacceptable risks to the extent that it is practicable (e.g., financially feasible). If it is not feasible to further reduce the risk, manufacturers may conduct a risk/benefit analysis to determine if the medical benefits of the intended use outweigh the residual risk.

In contrast, the ALAP approach does not allow manufacturers to consider practical and financial concerns when assessing whether they should further reduce a risk. Instead, manufacturers should explore opportunities to reduce all risks. Examples of cases in which manufacturers no longer need to reduce a risk include: (1) no additional risk controls exist that could further reduce the risk and (2) the manufacturer has implemented an effective risk control, and the risk cannot be mitigated by more than one risk control. As a result, manufacturers striving to meet EU regulatory expectations should demonstrate that they reduced all risks to as low as possible, despite the potential additional burden of doing so.

Additionally, the EU version of ISO 14971 indicates that manufacturers should not cite Instructions for Use and training as risk reduction measures in their overall risk estimations. Rather, the EU version calls upon manufacturers to focus on other design modifications to reduce risk, usually by reducing the likelihood of a use error as opposed to the severity of harm that could arise due to the use error.

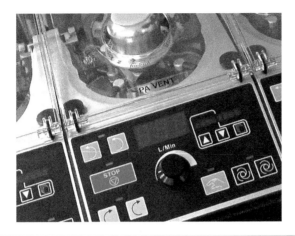

FIGURE 5.4   Ventilator includes a design-based risk mitigation, an emergency stop button.

Risk control—Process in which decisions are made and measures implemented by which risks are reduced to, or maintained within, specified levels.

The common way to control or reduce risk is to change a design so as to eliminate a hazard (e.g., sharp edge) or put a guard in place. Other risk controls (aka risk control measures), which are generally considered to be weaker than design changes and guards, include adding a warning and training people to avoid the hazard (Figure 5.4).

Residual risk—Risk remaining after risk control measures have been taken.

The concept of residual risk recognizes that risk cannot always be eliminated without having a negative effect on a given medical device's functional effectiveness. For example, there might never be a means to protect a surgeon from inadvertently cutting herself with an exposed scalpel tip, even if the device has a blade retraction feature to protect against such harm when the device is not in use. Opinions vary on the degree to which practicality, particularly with regard to the cost of implementing further safety measures, should factor into accepting a given level of residual risk (see Sidebar 5.1).

6

Types of Use Errors

There are many ways to categorize errors. What you find to be the most useful way depends on how simple or complicated you want to make things, and what you are trying to accomplish. In this chapter, we review some of the basic categorization schemes (i.e., taxonomies).

PERCEPTION, COGNITION, AND ACTION ERRORS

Here is the perception, cognition, and action organizing scheme discussed in IEC 62366-1:2015[*]:

Perception errors—Cases in which stimuli produced by a medical device do not register with the user (e.g., an alarm is too soft to be heard over the ambient noise) or are misperceived (e.g., the number "3" is perceived as an "8") (Figure 6.1). Perception errors can be tied not only to hearing and sight, but also to the senses of touch (feeling a button click), smell (detecting the odor of leaking insulin), and taste (tasting the flavor of an inhaled medication that contacts the tongue). You cannot observe another person making this kind of error, but that person can (1) describe such an error or (2) take incorrect

---

[*] IEC 62366-1:2015. "Medical Devices—Part 1: Application of Usability Engineering to Medical Devices."

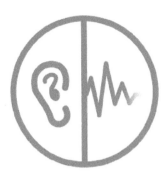

FIGURE 6.1 Perception errors are cases in which stimuli produced by a medical device do not register with the user.

actions or fail to take necessary actions that reveal it. For example, you can observe a person who has high-frequency hearing loss (presbycusis) fail to react to a high-frequency alarm.

Cognition errors—Cases in which the user does not remember something important (e.g., forgets to release a blood line clamp) or draws the wrong conclusion based on incomplete or flawed knowledge (e.g., decides to deliver an intravenous injection when a drug should be delivered via intramuscular injection) (Figure 6.2). Similar to a perception error, you cannot observe another person making this kind of error, but you can infer it for the same reasons stated before. For example, you can observe a pharmacist add too much diluent to a lyophilized drug (dry power) due to a mental math error.

Action errors—Cases in which the user does something—normally observable—that is incorrect (e.g., presses the wrong button) or is somehow prevented from completing a necessary step (e.g., being unable to apply enough force to get two components to connect properly) (Figure 6.3).

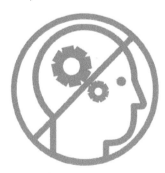

FIGURE 6.2 Cognition errors are cases in which the user does not remember something important or draws the wrong conclusion based on incomplete or flawed knowledge.

FIGURE 6.3   Action errors are cases when a user performs an incorrect action or does not perform a necessary step.

Note that IEC 62366-1:2015 uses the term "use error" in an intentionally narrow manner. It states:

> By the definition of this standard, a use error occurs at the "action" stage of this interaction cycle. This implies that errors that occur in the stage of perception (e.g., misreading a display) or at the stage of cognition (e.g., miscalculating a sum) are not considered use errors. Errors in perception and errors in cognition are rather considered contributing factors to or causes of use errors.[*]

This way of thinking about use errors makes some practical sense from a risk control standpoint. No harm can arise directly from someone failing to hear an alarm or making a mental math mistake. Harm can only arise from a user taking the wrong action or failing to take a necessary action. For example, not hearing an alarm could lead to the use error of not responding to the alarm, and not performing a mental calculation correctly could lead to the use error of delivering too little drug because the selected volume was too dilute. So, keep in mind that, from an IEC standard perspective, a use error occurs in the course of using a medical device, not just perceiving a stimuli or thinking about what to do.

IEC 62366-1:2015 goes further to characterize use errors as being related to normal versus abnormal use of a medical device. Normal use is equated to correct use, which in turn means that the user is operating the device as the manufacturer intended. The situation of a nurse using an intravenous infusion pump in an intensive care unit to hydrate a patient is considered normal or correct use. On the other hand, the scenario in which a layperson

---

[*] IEC 62366-1:2015. "Medical Devices—Part 1: Application of Usability Engineering to Medical Devices," Definition 3.21, "Use Error," p. 23.

SIDEBAR 6.1   THE SWISS CHEESE MODEL

James Reason and Dante Orlandella are credited with the swiss cheese model, which presents a particularly assessable way to think about accidents. Applying their model to a medical device accident (aka adverse event), the slices of cheese represent multiple efforts to prevent an accident, such as creating a user interface that reflects good human factors engineering, safeguards to prevent exposure to hazards that cannot be removed, warnings to alert users to take precautions, and instructions to guide safe interactions. The holes in the cheese slices represent limitations and shortcomings in the preventive measures. The arrow passing though the aligned holes depicts how some use errors might occur due to inadequacies in the preventive measures, thereby causing an accident—an injury or death (Figure 6.4).

uses the same device at home to deliver an antibiotic might be considered abnormal use because the pump was not intended to be used that way. The boundary between normal and abnormal use might be in question due to differing views about the limits of a manufacturer's responsibility to recognize use scenarios that might occur despite stated limits on a device's use (i.e., off-label use).

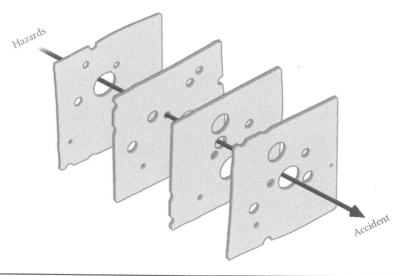

FIGURE 6.4   Swiss cheese model.

SLIPS, LAPSES, AND MISTAKES

Interestingly, IEC 62366:2007 formerly categorized errors in a different manner that was not so closely tied to the now-prevalent means of analyzing tasks by studying the flow of perception, cognition, and action as described previously. Matching the error categorization scheme presented in the popular book *The Design of Everyday Things*,* it placed use errors into these categories:

Slip—Cases in which the user's action does not match his or her intent. Intending to load a syringe with 30 mL of a drug, but inexplicably loading it with 60 mL is a slip, or what some people might call a mental slip. A user might be startled by a slip, having no idea why he or she did "such a stupid thing." Or the user might not notice a slip at all.

Lapse—Cases in which the user forgets to perform a necessary action. Forgetting to open a clamp on a dialysis machine's fluid line is a lapse. It is not necessarily an observable event but is detectable if you know what action should be performed and observe that it has not been done.

Mistake—Cases in which the user acts (or withholds action) deliberately but incorrectly. Deliberately connecting a gas line (e.g., oxygen) to an intravenous access port, misjudging the line to be one conveying a fluid (e.g., dextrose 5% in water), is a mistake.

---

* Norman, D. 1990. *The Design of Everyday Things*. New York: Doubleday Business.

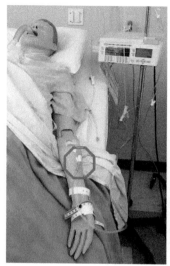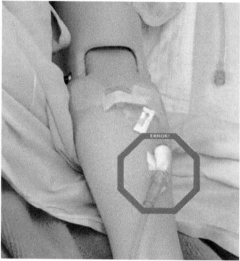

FIGURE 6.5 Simulated case in which a gas line is connected to a needleless IV port as depicted in the Medical Device Safety Calendar 2009, published by FDA. (Available at http://www.fda.gov/downloads/MedicalDevices/Safety/AlertsandNotices/UCM134873.pdf.)

Figure 6.5 depicts how a nurse could erroneously connect a gas line to a needleless IV port. This use error is very likely a mistake according to the preceding definitions because the nurse's action was deliberate even though it was wrong. The use error is not likely a slip because the erroneous action proceeded as intended. Moreover, the use error is not likely a lapse because the nurse did not suffer a memory failure per se. You could say that the nurse forgot that gas lines should not be connected to an IV access, but this is unlikely because such a connection defies basic safe practices. It is more likely that the nurse mistook the gas line to be a fluid line, given that both can appear clear.

ERRORS OF COMMISSION AND OMISSION

Another way to think about use errors is to divide them into the following two types:

> **Error of commission**—Cases in which someone performs an incorrect action. For example:
> + Pressing the wrong key on a keypad
> + Applying too much blood to a test strip (Figure 6.6)
> + Inserting batteries into a device backward

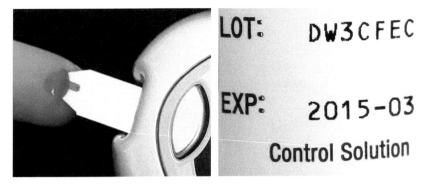

LOT: DW3CFEC

EXP: 2015-03

Control Solution

FIGURE 6.6 An error of commission is to apply too much blood to a blood glucose meter's test strip (left). An error of omission is to fail to inspect the test strip's expiration date and thus use an expired strip (right).

Error of omission—Cases in which someone did not act when he or she should have. For example:
+ Not pressing the "Enter" key after entering information into a data entry field
+ Not exhaling before taking a puff from an inhaler
+ Not wiping a Luer-type connector with an alcohol swab before attaching a needleless syringe to it

SAFETY-RELATED AND NON-SAFETY-RELATED USE ERRORS

Yet another way to categorize use errors has arisen as medical device developers have distinguished use errors that occur in usability tests. The dividing line pertains to an error's safety relevance.

Safety-related use error—Use errors that could cause harm (i.e., they pose a risk). For example:
+ Continuing to use a surgical instrument after it touches a non-sterile surface. Doing so could infect the surgical site.
+ Touching the patient at the moment an automated external defibrillator delivers a shock. Doing so could shock the caregiver in addition to the patient.
+ Not cleansing a nebulizer's breathing tubes after use. As a result, bacteria could grow in the tube and infect the user's respiratory tract during the next treatment.
Non-safety-related use error—Use errors that do not cause harm (i.e., they do not pose a risk). For example:

✦ Discarding a reusable pen-injector that still contains plenty of drug. The consequence might only be material waste and inconvenience.

✦ Pressing the "Clear" key instead of the "Enter" key after typing the patient's name into a data entry field. The consequence might only be waste of time, presuming that the use error does not cause a detrimental delay in therapy.

Some manufacturers go so far as to separate safety-related use errors into subcategories of those that pose high risk and those that pose low risk according to the associated risk analysis. They make this distinction to separate use errors they believe warrant root cause analysis and might require further risk control measures versus not requiring them.

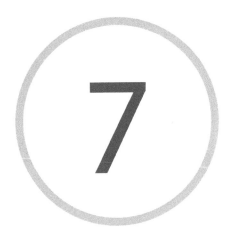

Detecting Use Errors

DETECTING USE ERRORS DURING USABILITY TESTS

Usability testing is the gold standard method to identify a medical device's interactive strengths and shortcomings. Use errors that occur during one or more test sessions signal opportunity for device improvement. Close calls, difficulties, slow task performance, and participants' negative criticism are also important signals.

Ahead of a usability test, you should determine what constitutes correct versus incorrect task performance. An appropriate first step is to identify all expected actions required to complete each task, based perhaps on the results of a task analysis. You should also make a list of all use errors appearing in a use-related risk analysis (see definition in Chapter 5). You can combine the list of expected actions and potential use errors to create tools, such as a use error checklist, for documenting task performance during usability test sessions.

Use error checklists can be paper-based and/or computer-based. Digital alternatives include a Microsoft Excel spreadsheet or specialized data logging software, such as the popular Morae® by TechSmith Corporation. These digital options enable data analysts to prepare specially-configured data collection tools that can reduce workload during test sessions. For example, prepopulated picklists enable data analysts to quickly select an anticipated use error rather than typing it in from scratch.

SIDEBAR 7.1   SAMPLE USE ERROR CHECKLIST

A paper-based use error checklist can list expected actions and anticipated potential use errors (often denoted "UE"). For example, the use error checklist used during a summative usability test of an inhaler might appear as follows:

Task 1: Use inhaler to deliver dose

_____ Remove inhaler cap

[UE] User does not remove cap

_____ Shake inhaler for at least 10 seconds
[UE] User does not shake inhaler
[UE] User shakes inhaler for less than 10 seconds

_____ Exhale fully
[UE] User does not exhale fully
[UE] User exhales into inhaler

_____ Place mouthpiece in mouth
[UE] User does not form tight seal with lips around mouthpiece

_____ Press inhaler canister and inhale mist
[UE] User does not press inhaler canister fully
[UE] ≥1-second delay between canister press and inhalation

_____ Hold breath for at least 5 seconds
[UE] User does not hold breath after inhaling
[UE] User holds breath for less than 5 seconds

_____ Replace inhaler cap
[UE] User does not replace cap

The test administrator should check off each step on the paper-based checklist as the participant completes it and circle the relevant use error if the participant commits it. The test administrator should also capture any unanticipated use errors that were not originally listed in the use error checklist by writing a detailed description of the error that occurred. A comparable checklist should be developed for each task in a summative usability test. In some cases, use error checklists are also used during formative usability tests.

In addition to looking for anticipated use errors, usability test personnel should also be on the lookout for unforeseen (i.e., unanticipated) use errors. Despite having anticipated and observed what might seem to be all potential use errors over the course of early analysis and testing, unforeseen use errors are surprisingly common, even at later stages of testing. Usability test personnel should confer frequently throughout the test session to ensure that all test team members have recognized and debriefed about any unanticipated use errors.

Detecting some use errors, such as installing a component (e.g., filter, battery, reservoir) backwards, is straightforward because the use error is readily apparent and easy to observe during a test session. That said, rapid task performance and/or an imperfect view of the "action" might prove to be an obstacle to real-time error detection. In such cases, you can perform a post-test review of close-up and/or slow-motion video of user–device interactions to detect any use errors that occurred but escaped initial detection.

SIDEBAR 7.2   DETECTING USE ERRORS BY REVIEWING USABILITY TEST VIDEO

Sometimes video review is necessary to enable usability test personnel to detect certain use errors. For example, imagine the scenario of a usability test conducted to assess an intranasal drug delivery device (i.e., nasal spray) that requires the user to split the dose evenly between both nostrils. Ideally, you would record close-up, high-resolution video of nasal administration and review the video after the test sessions to determine how much drug the participants delivered to each nostril, whether the participants split the dose evenly, or if they committed the use error of delivering most of the drug into one nostril and almost no drug into the other nostril.

Some use errors defy detection via real-time observation or video review, simply because they cannot be seen. In such cases, you might be able to identify these use errors by waiting for other events to transpire. For example, a nurse programming an enteral pump (a device that delivers liquid food through a nasogastric or percutaneous feeding tube) might mistakenly enter a flow rate of 500 mL/hour when she meant to enter 400 mL/hour. She might have inadvertently pressed the keypad's "5" key when she was aiming for the "4" key, but you might not immediately recognize this as an unintended result if 400 and 500 mL/hour are both legitimate inputs, independent of user intent. If the higher rate was not an obvious error in the given use scenario, or if the nurse had momentarily turned the pump's screen out of view, you would not be able to detect the error immediately. Instead, you might detect the error only when the nurse returns to the pump's home screen where the rate is visible, for example. During follow-up interviews, the nurse might spontaneously mention the error, or she might only recollect or mention it when you ask her if she recalled making any mistakes.

DETECTING USE ERRORS DURING CLINICAL STUDIES

There are at least a few ways to detect use errors when a device is being used during a clinical study. One way is to observe users in the same manner as one would during a usability test. However, such observations are likely to be less productive because people are using the device in routine ways and might never perform infrequent tasks or face rare malfunctions (e.g., pump failure, screen failure, and automatic shutdown due to overheating). By comparison, usability testing enables you to introduce unusual use scenarios and simulate component failures. Still, observations in a clinical setting might be worthwhile to capture the most realistic use scenarios.

Another way to detect use errors that occur when a device is in clinical use is to ask clinicians and/or patients to report use errors, perhaps by keeping a paper-based or digital diary. In addition to documenting use errors that they commit, you could also ask clinicians to keep a diary of the use errors that they observe their patients commit.

A shortcoming of the diary approach is that there might be gaps between the actual events that occurred and the errors recorded in the diary by the clinician or patient. For example, a clinician might be unaware she committed an error, so she did not record it in the diary. You can also interview users about their experience using the device over the course of the clinical study and ask if they recall making any mistakes using the device. These interviews can occur over the phone or in person and can be conducted one-on-one or as a group discussion with several clinical study participants.

The diary-keeping approach may capture even more use errors if people faithfully report them on a daily or at least weekly basis, whereas a single interview near the end of a clinical study might cause users to forget past use errors or at least the associated details.

Here are some use errors that participants in a clinical study might report in a diary about their experience using a home dialysis machine

✦ Dropped the disposable tubing set on the floor, and then had to throw it away because it was contaminated.
✦ Did not disinfect hands before handling the tubing set.
✦ Used an expired bag of dialysate solution.
✦ Connected incorrect dialysate solution bag (of the wrong concentration) to tubing set.
✦ Entered the wrong therapy time when setting up the dialysis machine, thereby shortening the amount of time the dialysate solution remained in the peritoneal cavity during each cycle.

DETECTING USE ERRORS DURING THE DEVICE'S LIFE CYCLE

A combination of requirements presented in ISO 13485:2003[*] and ISO 14971:2007[†] calls upon manufacturers to perform post-market surveillance of their medical devices. This means manufacturers must vigilantly check information sources for indications that their devices pose a greater risk to users than anticipated and accepted when the devices received regulatory clearance. In other words, they have to monitor for events during which a use error led to or almost led to an adverse event. Such events might trigger a recall or other remedial action.

FDA's HFE guidance[‡] to industry lists the following resources where one might find reports of use errors leading to adverse events.

✦ FDA's Manufacturer and User Facility Device Experience (MAUDE) database
✦ FDA's Medical Device Reporting (MDR) Program Search
✦ FDA's Adverse Event Reporting Data Files
✦ FDA's MedSun: Medical Product Safety Network

---

[*] ISO 13485:2003. "Medical Devices—Quality Management Systems—Requirements for Regulatory Purposes."
[†] ISO 14971:2007. "Medical Devices—Application of Risk Management to Medical Devices."
[‡] "Draft Guidance for Industry and Food and Drug Administration Staff—Applying Human Factors and Usability Engineering to Optimize Medical Device Design" (document issued June 22, 2011).

+ CDRH Medical Device Recalls
+ CDRH Alerts and Notices (Medical Devices)
+ CDRH Public Health Notifications
+ ECRI's Medical Device Safety Reports
+ The Institute of Safe Medical Practices (ISMP's) Medication Safety Alert Newsletters
+ The Joint Commission's Sentinel Events

Note that some of the reports might not explicitly state that a use error led to the given adverse event because the reporter did not view the event from an HFE perspective. However, close analysis of such reports often supports the conclusion that one or more use errors occurred. Importantly, most use errors are not reported. As such, while these reports are a valuable tool for identifying use errors, you should not assume the reports are an accurate indication of a use error's frequency of occurrence.

SIDEBAR 7.3   ISO 13485:2003 AND ISO 14971:2007

ISO 13485:2003 ("Medical Devices—Quality Management Systems—Requirements for Regulatory Purposes") calls upon manufacturers to establish a quality management system. It implicitly requires manufacturers to implement a risk management process. This in turn calls for the assessment and reduction of use-related risks and, therefore, performing root cause analysis as a basis for identifying opportunities to lower risks.

ISO 14971:2007 ("Medical Devices—Application of Risk Management to Medical Devices") explains that performing post-market surveillance should be an element of a manufacturer's quality management system. Manufacturers should establish a procedure for obtaining, reviewing, and responding (if necessary) to this data collected during post-market surveillance. The type of post-market surveillance can vary by product and should be described and justified in a product's risk management plan.

We discuss these standards more in Chapter 4.

A straightforward means to identify use errors that occur in the field is to interview people who have filed adverse event reports, mirroring how you would interview usability test participants who committed a use error (see Chapter 8). However, access to such individuals can be complicated by two primary factors. One factor is that a manufacturer might learn about a use error well after it occurred, in which case the individual(s) involved might have changed jobs or might not recall important details of the event. Another factor is that a use error might have led to a harm, which subsequently triggered legal posturing that blocks access to the individual(s) involved.

Even if it is not possible to conduct a post-event interview for the aforementioned reasons, you can still conduct a root cause analysis of the event using the method we outlined in Chapter 2.

SIDEBAR 7.4   AAMI TECHNICAL INFORMATION REPORT ON POST-MARKET SURVEILLANCE

In 2014, the Association for the Advancement of Medical Instrumentation (AAMI) published AAMI TIR50:2014 "Technical Information Report, Post-Market Surveillance of Use Error Management."

PURPOSE[*]

This document addresses the issue of use error detection for medical devices from the clinical, manufacturer, patient, user, and regulatory perspectives. The goal is to provide guidance on how these individuals can best collect, assess, and leverage postmarket use error data to mitigate product risk, and to improve product safety and usability.

The technical information report points to the following information resources when performing post-market surveillance, including researching the cause of a use error that led to an adverse event:

- Relevant vigilance reports
- Joint Commission sentinel event alerts
- Incident reports
- Adverse event reports (e.g., MDRs submitted to the FDA)
- Customer complaints
- MedWatch data
- Closed claim data
- Post-market surveillance data (e.g., CAPA—corrective action and preventive action)
- Precursor analysis
- Use of critical incident analysis techniques
- Structured interviews with users who have experienced problems with the device

---

[*] Available at http://my.aami.org/store/detail.aspx?id=TIR50-PDF

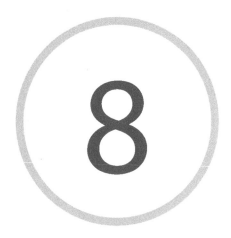

Interviewing Users to Determine Root Causes

INTRODUCTION

Usability test participants can be your greatest ally in the search for the root causes of use errors. All you have to do is ask them—in the proper manner, of course—why they think they made mistakes. Their responses serve as valuable inputs toward forming hypotheses on the most likely root causes.

Let's set the scene. There is a 30-participant, summative usability test underway. This particular test session's participant is a nurse who has worked in a large teaching hospital's pediatric intensive care unit for the past seven years. The nurse has the requisite advanced life support (ALS) training and has hands-on patient care experience. She also has experience using a wide array of medical devices, including many types of ventilators (artificial breathing machines). The task at hand is to set up a ventilator to deliver respiratory support to a one-year-old child (represented by

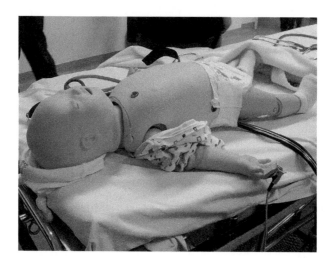

FIGURE 8.1   Sample of a pediatric mannequin. (Photo courtesy of Liam Skoda. Accessed from https://commons.wikimedia.org/wiki/File:Simbaby.jpg)

an advanced pediatric mannequin in this simulated usability test case) (Figure 8.1).

The task goes smoothly until the participant neglects to switch the ventilator from "adult" to "pediatric" mode. In a real use scenario, this mistake could lead to a catastrophic lung injury (e.g., major hemorrhaging due to being overpressurized), so it should be counted as a critical use error. The pressing question in this hypothetical case is: Why did the nurse make the mistake? In other words, what is the mistake's root cause?

The usability test team running the session, and perhaps even the session observers, might already have a couple of root causes in mind, perhaps because they have seen the error before and linked it to a particular user interface design shortcoming. Maybe they think the root causes are that (1) the ventilator does not require the user to select a ventilation mode, but rather uses the most recent setting and (2) the ventilation mode indicator is relatively inconspicuous because it is embedded in a rather dense set of information and displayed in undifferentiated, 10-point text. Regardless of their certitude about the mistake's root cause(s), they should ask the test participant to speculate about the mistake's root cause.

The test participant might suggest a plausible root cause, but this is not always the case. Some people just are not very good at diagnosing their mistakes, so a given test participant might cite an implausible root cause, blame himself or herself (see Chapter 9), or state, "I have no idea." Experienced usability test specialists are loath to accept the latter response and will endeavor to coax a more helpful response.

The following sections describe important considerations for interviewing test participants and strategies for conducting productive interviews when seeking to identity a use error's root cause.

INTERVIEW TIMING

There is a right time and a wrong time to ask a test participant about mistakes. Optimal timing depends on the type of usability test. You have more flexibility when conducting a formative usability test, the purpose of which is to learn about a device's user interface design strengths and opportunities for improvement. Summative usability testing is a more rigid process that usually constrains when you can ask follow-up questions.

INTERVIEWING PARTICIPANTS DURING FORMATIVE USABILITY TESTS

In most cases, we find it more productive to ask a formative usability test participant about a mistake shortly after it occurs, when the participant has a fresh sense for what happened. Here is a hypothetical dialog that illustrates how you can ask follow-up questions in the moment:

> *Test participant:* Oh no. I think I did something wrong. This isn't right at all.
>
> *Test administrator:* What happened?
>
> *Test participant:* I think I programmed the pump wrong. I programmed the secondary infusion at the primary infusion's rate. That's a bad mistake.
>
> *Test administrator:* What do you think caused the mistake?
>
> *Test participant:* Hmmm. Not certain. Maybe because the primary and secondary rate fields look similar. But, I should have read it more carefully. You can blame me.
>
> *Test administrator:* Tell me more about the similar appearance of the fields and why it concerns you.
>
> *Test participant:* Sure. The fields look the same. Even the labels are similar: P-infusion and S-infusion. There's a single letter distinguishing them and not everyone is going to pick up on the subtle difference.
>
> *Test administrator:* Any other comments?
>
> *Test participant:* Everything else is the same. Rate. Volume. You can be plugging in numbers in the wrong field without knowing it. There really should be a confirmation that asks you to check that you have set the primary and secondary the way you want them to be set.
>
> *Test administrator:* OK. Thank you for that feedback. Let's move on.

Note that the sample dialog brings the task at hand to a temporary stop, which might influence how the test participant proceeds to correct the problem and perform subsequent tasks. So, there is a clear trade-off between obtaining fresh insights into root causes of use errors and possibly changing how test participants interact with a given device.

During a formative usability test, one can rationalize interrupting the task with questions because the goal is to identify opportunities for design improvement. An alternative to reflecting on events immediately after they occur is to wait until the end of the task—an expected closure point. This approach encourages a more natural task flow, but complicates root cause identification if a participant commits multiple use errors during a single extended task, or if significant time has elapsed since the use error occurred.

INTERVIEWING PARTICIPANTS DURING SUMMATIVE USABILITY TESTS

Our practice, derived from FDA guidance on the topic, is to ask a summative usability test participant about a mistake in the least intrusive manner possible. Typically, this means holding our questions until the participant completes the task at hand, or perhaps even a series of tasks that normally proceed in an uninterrupted sequence.

The conclusion of a task is a natural "break in the action" and, therefore, an opportunity to discuss how the task progressed without interrupting the normal work flow. In other words, we allow for test participants to make mistakes and continue working through the given task and related follow-on tasks. This approach prevents us from influencing the participant's task performance.

During follow-up discussions, we will ask the objective question: Do you recall making any mistakes while performing the tasks? If the test participant recalls making one or more mistakes, it is time to ask more specific questions. Here is a sample dialog that illustrates how you might ask follow-up questions after some time has passed since the mistake occurred, and after initiating the discussion with a general inquiry about mistakes:

> *Test administrator:* Do you recall making any mistakes while performing the tasks?
>
> *Test participant:* Yes. I got the primary and secondary infusion programs reversed.
>
> *Test administrator:* Tell me more about that.
>
> *Test participant:* I confused them. I plugged in the primary infusion data in the field that is supposed to be for the secondary infusion.
>
> *Test administrator:* What do you think caused the mistake?

This dialog might follow the same productive pattern presented earlier for a formative usability test. Alternatively, given that several minutes might have passed since the use error occurred, the dialog might continue down a less productive path, as follows:

Test participant: I don't exactly remember why I made that mistake.
Test administrator: Speculate if you can.
Test participant: I think I was just working too fast. Sometimes you have to slow down and carefully examine what you are doing.
Test administrator: Rather than blaming yourself, can you suggest anything about the device that might have caused the mistake?
Test participant: Not really. I needed to slow down.

You can see from this example and the prior one that delaying questions about root causes can interfere with a test participant's ability to cite plausible possibilities. But, this is considered a necessary trade-off—a regulators' mandate, really—considering that we want to avoid influencing task performance during a summative usability test.

What if the test participant does not recall making a mistake that actually occurred (you observed it)? After discussing all mistakes the participant recollects, you should then follow up on any other mistakes that occurred. Here is one more sample dialog that takes this course:

Test administrator: Do you recall making any other mistakes that we have not already discussed?
Test participant: No. I think we have covered them all.
Test administrator: Fair enough. My colleague and I noted a few other events I'd like to ask you about.
Test participant: Sure. Did I make some other mistakes?
Test administrator: We noticed that you placed the secondary infusion solution bag at the same height as the primary infusion bag, instead of placing the secondary bag higher than the primary bag. Can you comment on why you did that?
Test participant: OK. I see that I did that. That's obviously not correct. The secondary bag should be higher than the primary bag or you're not going to get the right flow.
Test administrator: What do you think caused the mistake?
Test participant: I thought I hung the secondary higher than the primary, but I see that I mixed up which bag is which. I think what caused my mistake is the way the pump made me review and confirm the programs for the primary and secondary infusion, but it never reminded me to confirm that the secondary infusion bag was hung

higher than the primary infusion. With so many other steps in the task, I must have forgotten that step.

Despite the value of having test participants suggest design modifications, such as during a formative usability test, it is inappropriate to solicit design suggestions from participants during a summative usability test. Summative usability testing should be focused on collecting data that will determine if the production-equivalent, final design is safe and effective, rather than take the more exploratory approach of inviting design suggestions after each task. A steady dialog about potential improvements could bias follow-on tasks. That said, FDA and perhaps some other regulators want summative usability tests to conclude with the general query (variants accepted): "Do you think the device is safe as is or does it need to be improved to ensure safe use?" It is fine if test participants spontaneously suggest design improvements when reflecting on a mistake. Just do not prompt test participants for such feedback after each discrete task or related series of tasks. Importantly, wait until the test participant has completed all tasks to ask the participant whether he or she thinks the device is safe as is.

INTERVIEW TIPS

The sample dialogs presented previously instantiate the following interview tips:

+ Ask simple, neutral, and objective questions.
+ Keep questions short. Let the test participant do most of the talking.
+ Invite participants to say more when you sense that there is more on their minds.
+ Seek clarification when participants make general or ambiguous statements.
+ Discourage participants from blaming themselves for mistakes. Invite them to consider the possibility that the device induced the mistakes.
+ Do not provide feedback on the quality of the participant's feedback, although, it may encourage productive subsequent dialog if you intermittently say, "Thank you for the feedback."

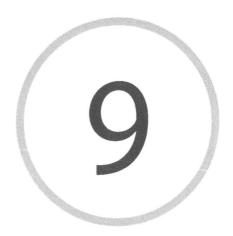

Perils of Blaming
Users for Use Errors

DON'T BLAME THE USER

There is an understandable tendency among people, particularly those who are not human factors specialists, to observe a use error that occurs during a usability test and conclude that it was the user's fault. After all, there can be no use error without a user. Viewed simplistically, a use error calls for someone to make a mistake of some sort; pressing the wrong button, assembling device components incorrectly, administering medication using an incorrect technique, or forgetting to click a "Confirm" button. As such, it is a natural tendency to blame the user for a mistake he or she committed—even more so if the person making judgments is intellectually, emotionally, and perhaps financially invested in the medical device performing satisfactorily (Figure 9.1).

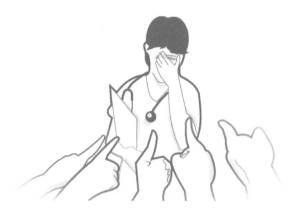

FIGURE 9.1   Avoid blaming the user.

The reality is that use errors involving a medical device are almost always induced by user interface design flaws (see Chapter 10). Small text leads to reading errors. Buttons with minimal travel and a "squishy" feel usually deprive users of the tactile feedback needed to be sure their button presses register. Confusing and unfamiliar names for software menu options lead users to select the wrong item. For some usability test observers, as well as folks who read usability test reports, this is, to use an Al Gore-ism, an *inconvenient truth*[*] and can be a bitter pill to swallow.

Now, we will digress. Indeed, people can make mistakes for absolutely no discernible reason. Psychologists call such events *blunders*. Some researchers estimate the rate at which human beings acting with care still blunder to be approximately 1%,[†] but it is heavily dependent on the nature of the associated task, the use environment, and other performance-shaping factors. Another term that may be used to describe a use error is *idiopathic*, meaning something that "arises spontaneously or from an unknown or obscure cause."[‡] Mental lapses, such as removing a sandwich from a plastic sandwich bag and throwing the sandwich in the trash instead of the bag, could be described as blunders and idiopathic errors.

But talk of blunders and idiopathic use errors is best set aside when searching for the root cause of medical device error, chiefly because almost all such errors can be traced to an underlying, design-related cause. We believe that this point—*that design flaws, not users, are usually the root causes of use errors*—should be a tenet of all root cause analysis of medical device use error.

---

[*] The term "inconvenient truth" was popularized in a 2006 film, called *An Inconvenient Truth,* featuring Al Gore.

[†] Kirwan, B. 1994. *A Guide to Practical Human Reliability Assessment.* Bristol, PA: Taylor & Francis.

[‡] Merriam-Webster dictionary. Accessed from http://www.merriam-webster.com/dictionary/idiopathic.

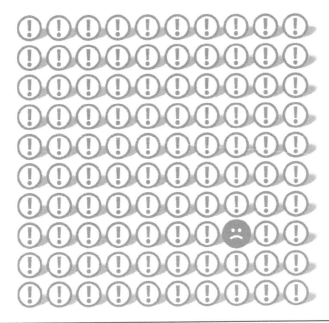

FIGURE 9.2   We suggest that 1 in 100 use errors is actually the user's fault.

Blaming the user for an error should be your last recourse. If you want to use our rule of thumb, which builds on the concept of a fundamental blunder rate, we suggest that only 1 in 100 use errors is purely the user's fault (Figure 9.2).

Still, some people will insist on blaming users for mistakes. In usability test observation and debriefing rooms, we've heard it all. "What an idiot!" "Nobody would do that in the real world!" "That's a once in a million mistake!"

Here are some of the ways people have tried to explain away use errors, paraphrased in the first person.

+ **Anxious**—That nurse seemed very nervous, which interfered with his ability to concentrate.
+ **Camera shy**—The adolescent said she was extremely camera shy. There's no question that her shyness distracted her from the task at hand. She'd have flown through the task if she had not been watched and video recorded.
+ **Careless**—The technician was the kind of person who doesn't think through what he is doing before acting. He's impulsive, if you ask me. And he didn't seem to care if he did things right or wrong.
+ **Disinterested**—The participant acted bored. Did you see how often he checked his watch? He didn't seem to recognize the importance of

operating the device correctly. That's not how people will do things in the real world.

+ **Disregarded instructions**—The physician paid no attention to the Instructions for Use. She didn't even take them out of the box. She even said that she hates to read instructions.

+ **Fatigued**—The nurse had already worked a 10-hour shift and then driven through heavy traffic to the usability test facility. So, she was hardly in any condition to give tasks her full attention. She would have aced the tasks if she was fresh.

+ **Forgetful**—The participant was trained to perform the task only two hours earlier. She obviously just forgot what she was taught. Makes you wonder if she has a serious memory problem.

+ **Inattentive**—The participant's mind seemed to drift in the middle of the task. She didn't seem at all focused.

+ **Low intelligence**—The guy obviously has low intelligence. He read and spoke very slowly, like something was wrong with him. He didn't seem to grasp even the basic concept of how to use the device.

+ **Negative attitude**—The technician clearly wanted to be elsewhere rather than participating in the test. I'm not sure why he didn't just cancel on us. He didn't seem to give the hands-on tasks much of an effort.

+ **Non-compliant**—The participant read the instructions that told him not to turn the device on before loading the cassette. But, he chose to turn the device on right away despite knowing he shouldn't. Who does that?

+ **Risk-taking**—I know this type of guy. He's the type who is comfortable taking risks. A real cowboy. He was not at all concerned about performing the task with the necessary precision.

+ **Rushed**—During the whole test session, the guy seemed to be rushing to get done and leave with his honorarium. He probably had to pick up his kids at daycare.

Some people will blame users for mistakes and be indignant—and perhaps even furious—if you place blame on a medical device's user interface design. You may disarm this tendency by counseling usability test observers about the reality that design shortcomings are the usual root causes of most use errors, and you should do so before testing begins. When approaching the task of root cause analysis, potentially working with a multidisciplinary team, establish a simple rule: Do not blame the user. Following this rule will lead you and others to look first and energetically for design-related root causes of use errors.

If you resort to blaming the user frequently, design-related root causes might go undiagnosed and leave user interface design flaws unresolved.

Furthermore, regulators who review your root cause analysis might lose confidence in your analysis because they recognize that design flaws, not people, are the root cause of most use errors, accepting that users are part of the failure mechanism. Only in rare instances does blaming the user uphold your credibility as an analyst, and it tends to legitimize the limited cases in which you do place blame on the user.

SIDEBAR 9.1   WHY WE MAKE MISTAKES

In the book *Why We Make Mistakes*, which is both informative and entertaining, Joseph Hallinan states, "If multiple people make the same mistake, then that should tell us something about the nature of the mistake being made: its cause probably isn't individual but systemic. Any systemic errors have their roots at a level *above* the individual. Which is why, when looking for the source of errors, it pays to look up and not down."[*]

Applying this view, so to speak, one might assess how workplace issues cause use errors involving a medical device. For example, a poorly conceived and executed training program could trigger use errors.

---

[*] Hallinan, J. 2009. *Why We Make Mistakes*. New York: Broadway Books, p. 191.

REPORTING TEST ARTIFACT AS A ROOT CAUSE OF USE ERROR

In some cases, usability test artifact (i.e., artificialities associated with conducting a simulation) can lead to use errors in a usability test. For example, a participant performing a simulated injection task on a simulated skin pad might skip the step of cleaning the injection site with an alcohol wipe because he considered it unnecessary to clean an inanimate surface that was not real skin. Alternatively, a participant might not verbalize that she would wash her hands before performing an injection because there is not a sink in the room.

As you can see from these examples, there are legitimate situations in which test artifact can lead to use errors. These situations indicate opportunities to revise the test method during future device testing. However, usability specialists would do well to consider all other potential causes of a use error before "blaming the test." For example, after observing several test participants discard a used, capped needle in the trash, a less experienced analyst might attribute this use error to the simulated use environment and assume that participants would take more care (and, therefore, discard the needle in a sharps container) if they performed the task in "real life." However, if the specialist conducts a thorough root cause analysis, he or she might identify a key user interface design flaw: the instruction sheet does not provide direction about where to discard the used needle, and it does not warn against discarding the used needle in the trash. As such, these participants did not realize that discarding the needle in the trash was a safety hazard and that they should instead discard it in a sharps container. Simply stated, you should consider root causes related to user interface design flaws before concluding that a test artifact led to a use error.

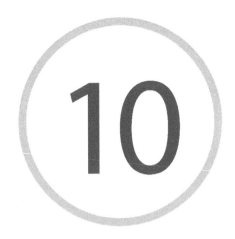

User Interface
Design Flaws
That Can Lead
to Use Error

INTRODUCTION

In Chapter 9, we discourage folks from blaming the user for making mistakes when operating a medical device. We assert that most use errors are induced by a medical device's hardware and software user interface design flaws and not by user ineptitude in various forms. Disbelievers need only to observe a few usability test sessions to witness the pattern of repeated use errors that particular user interface design flaws can induce if the device has not already been "scrubbed clean" of such flaws.

Sample user interface design flaws that we have observed to cause use errors include the following:

✦ Misleading or ambiguous wording that causes users to select the wrong menu option.

✦ A keypad that lacks an effective debounce algorithm (i.e., software designed to disregard an input that occurs very closely in time to a prior one) and, therefore, is vulnerable to unintended double key presses and the resulting data entry errors.

✦ A ventilator's air filter that can be inserted backward into its housing, thereby preventing proper airflow.

✦ A patient scale that displays units of measure in small text that is some distance from the associated data readout, thereby leading users to mistake a measurement made in pounds as one made in kilograms.

Some user interface design flaws can be detected through usability inspection methods such as a heuristic analysis.* Other flaws might become evident only when you conduct a usability test.

As you might expect, a particular user interface design flaw is unlikely to cause every test participant to err. For example, only a few people might commit a use error during a usability test involving 15, 30, 45, or even more participants. However, even if there is just one use error, that error warrants close examination to determine if there is a way to improve the user interface to eliminate the opportunity for it to occur, or at least to reduce its likelihood. This approach aligns with the general strategy applied in many engineering fields that calls for design solutions that eliminate hazards as the first order of business, followed by efforts to reduce the risk associated with hazards that cannot be eliminated.

Let's talk some more about the case of a single use error. Why would anyone get concerned about such a singularity, particularly if we presume that no medical device can ever be perfect?

Suppose one person commits a particular error during a usability test of a glucose meter involving 30 people. Now suppose the manufacturer places 20,000 devices into use and each device is used an average of four times a day. This scenario presents 80,000 opportunities for the use error to occur each day. Therefore, a persistent error rate of 1 in 30 would result in over 2,500 use errors per day. Granted, there are various reasons that the actual error rate might be much lower than suggested by the results of a test that focuses on initial ease of use, particularly because users are likely to learn how to operate their devices properly over time. But, if only 1% of the predicted use

---

* Nielsen, J. (1994). *Usability Inspection Methods.* New York: Wiley.

errors eventually lead to harm, there would still be 25 adverse events per day and over 9,000 per year.

Many of these adverse events would likely go unreported, which is why regulators estimate that use errors involving medical devices are causing much greater harm than indicated in such reporting systems as MAUDE—Manufacturer and User Facility Device Experience.[*]

If you buy into the logical case presented here, you will appreciate the intense focus that regulators now place on applying human factors engineering in medical device development and the level of effort that manufacturers must exert to comply with regulators' human factors engineering expectations. As shown previously, a single use error that occurs during a test can indicate the potential for hundreds or thousands occurring in the field.

Many use errors can be avoided by applying human factors engineering design principles in the course of user interface design. Reference literature such as ANSI/AAMI HE75:2009/(R)2013[†] is chock full of such design principles. Here is a wide-ranging sample of those found in the 460+ page document.[‡]

SECTION 21.4.11.3.C

Touch target spacing—In general, the centers of touch screen targets should be spaced 2.0 cm (0.8 inch) apart to help users avoid pressing the wrong target, but reduced spacing might be necessary to accommodate more targets on a small display.

SECTION 15.4.5

Alarms—The key information that the alarm signals have to convey is what the source of the problem is, what the problem is, what needs to be done (if possible), and how urgent it is. In other words, the user has to know the location of the problem, the cause of the problem, and what action is necessary to address it.

SECTION 23.4.2.2.B

Workstations—Workstations should require users to confirm critical and irreversible machine functions, giving users time to detect and

---

[*] MAUDE—Manufacturer and User Facility Device Experience. Available at http://www. accessdata.fda.gov/scripts/cdrh/cfdocs/cfmaude/search.cfm. The website states: "The MAUDE database houses medical device reports submitted to the FDA by mandatory reporters (manufacturers, importers and device user facilities) and voluntary reporters such as health care professionals, patients and consumers."

[†] ANSI/AAMI HE75:2009/(R)2013. "Human Factors Engineering—Design of Medical Devices."

[‡] Reproduced with permission from AAMI.

correct slips and mistakes that could waste time, waste resources (e.g., a tubing set), and cause property damage and possible harm to the user or patient.

SECTION 21.4.6.6

Line spacing—Lines of text should be spaced far enough apart to ensure that a gap of at least one pixel or greater exists between the ascending letterforms (e.g., bdfhklt) and descending letterforms (e.g., gjpqy). Additional space (i.e., leading) between lines will make text more readable by avoiding a crowded appearance.

SECTION 24.3.2.1

Edges, corners, and pinch points—Sharp edges, corners, and other mechanical features that can injure users or patients (e.g., potential pinch points) should be avoided. For example, a diagnostic electrocardiograph cart with sharp edges could cause avoidable patient injury if it were to tip over on the patient or be pushed firmly against the patient's bed.

These guidelines may be used in the following ways:

✦ Convert the guidelines into user interface design specifications to develop designs that are resistant to use error.
✦ Employ the guidelines as user interface design heuristics in the course of a design inspection.
✦ Cite the guidelines as good HFE practice when documenting the root causes of use errors that occur during a usability test (see Chapter 11).

SIDEBAR 10.1   PRIORITIES FOR CONTROLLING OR MITIGATING USE-RELATED RISKS

FDA's human factors engineering guidance* states:
    The following list presents the order of overall priority for applying strategies to control or mitigate risks of use-related hazards.

---

* "Draft Guidance for Industry and Food and Drug Administration Staff—Applying Human Factors and Usability Engineering to Optimize Medical Device Design" (issued June 22, 2011).

1. *Modify the device design to remove a hazard or reduce its consequences:* For example, making the user interface intuitive and ensuring that critical information is effectively communicated to the user can reduce the likelihood of or eliminate certain use-related hazards. If hazards cannot be eliminated, the design should, to the extent possible, reduce their likelihood and the severity of any consequences.

2. *Make the user interface, including its operating logic, error tolerant:* When errors occur during device use, such as users pressing an adjacent key on a keypad, the device should act to preclude a hazardous outcome. Safety mechanisms such as physical safety guards, shielded controls, or software or hardware interlocks will make the design more tolerant of errors that users might make.

3. *Alert users to the hazard:* When neither design nor safety features will eliminate a use-related hazard or adequately mitigate the consequences, the device should detect the condition and provide an adequate warning signal to users.

4. *Develop written procedures and training for safe operation:* If it is impossible to eliminate hazards through any of the previous strategies, or to enhance other control or mitigation strategies, then written procedures, labeling enhancements, and training for safe operation are the remaining options.

SIDEBAR 10.2   IEC 62366-1:2015,[*] SUBCLAUSE 4.1.2

RISK CONTROL as it relates to USER INTERFACE design

If practicable, the MEDICAL DEVICE should be designed to be inherently safe. If this is not practicable, then protective measures such as barriers or actively informing the USER are appropriate. The least preferred protective measure is information for SAFETY such as a written warning or contraindication. The MANUFACTURER should document the rationale for the option chosen in the USABILITY ENGINEERING FILE.

[*] IEC 62366-1:2015. "Medical Devices—Part 1: Application of Usability Engineering to Medical Devices."

Now, we have established that use errors can lead to harm and that use errors usually trace back to user interface design deficiencies, to which one could refer more politely as "shortcomings." The rest of this chapter describes an array of these user interface design shortcomings, many of which we have observed lead to use errors. Considering all the ways that a particular user interface could be compromised, our collection is just the "tip of the iceberg" of possibilities.

You will see that many of the following flaws are also cited as the entire or partial root cause of the use errors analyzed in Chapter 12.

GENERAL USER INTERFACE DESIGN FLAW EXAMPLES

INADEQUATE FEEDBACK (OR DELAYED FEEDBACK)

✦ *Problem:* Users can become confused and/or induced to err by user interfaces that provide little, delayed, or no feedback through the available channels (e.g., audio, visual, and tactile).

✦ *Sample use error:* User does not believe that a device registered a button press because he or she did not feel a click, so the user presses the button again.

✦ *Consequence:* The double button press initially activates and then deactivates a function.

INSUFFICIENT USER SUPPORT

✦ *Problem:* Users struggle to operate a device for the first few times because it provides a limited amount of user support. Specifically, the Instructions for Use are terse to a fault, the computer-based device has no online help, screens do not include informative prompts, and there is no Quick Reference Guide.

✦ *Sample use error:* User does not remove ancillary items from a patient's hospital bed before initiating a baseline patient weight measurement.

✦ *Consequence:* Future weight readings are distorted because the initial reading was artificially high. Clinicians conclude that the patient has experienced a significant weight loss and proceed with unnecessary therapies to address it.

SIMILAR NAMES

✦ *Problem:* Users mistake similar items that have similar looking and/ or sounding names.

✦ *Sample use error:* User programs an intravenous infusion pump to deliver Dobutamine instead of Dopamine.

✦ *Consequence:* Patient receives wrong drug.

Too Many Procedural Steps

✦ *Problem:* A procedure that includes many steps can lead users to forget and, therefore, skip an essential step.

✦ *Sample use error:* User forgets to check the expiration date when preparing to deliver an injection using a prefilled syringe.

✦ *Consequence:* User administers an expired drug, which might have negative health effects (e.g., ineffectiveness at treating the medical condition).

HARDWARE USER INTERFACE DESIGN FLAW EXAMPLES

Closely Spaced Buttons

✦ *Problem:* Closely spaced buttons, such as those found on a relatively small numeric entry pad, can induce users to press the wrong button by accident, typically because the user's finger extends beyond the target button and actuates a nearby button.

✦ *Sample use error:* User unintentionally presses the "8" rather than the intended "5" button, thereby entering the wrong flow rate into a drug pump.

✦ *Consequence:* Patient receives the wrong dose of medication.

Complex Connection

✦ *Problem:* Users can take more time than expected or available to connect components that have unfamiliar interlocking features or simply do not readily connect.

✦ *Sample use error:* User takes a long time to connect a communication cable to an implanted therapy device, principally because he or she does not recognize the need to align markings on the components to be connected.

✦ *Consequence:* The consequence is delayed therapy delivery.

Display Glare

✦ *Problem:* Glare can impede users' ability to read a display because the displayed information is partially or completely washed out by reflected light.

✦ *Sample use error:* User does not see a prompt to log if a blood glucose reading was taken before or after a meal.

✦ *Consequence:* User does not complete a key operation enabling effective diabetes management (Figure 10.1).

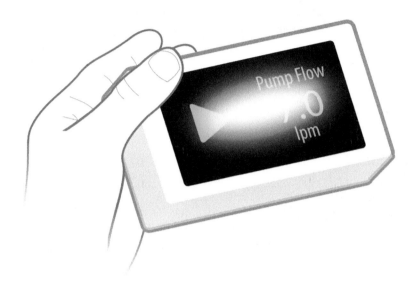

FIGURE 10.1 Glare impedes the user's ability to read the pump's display.

INAUDIBLE ALARM

✦ *Problem:* Users might not detect an alarm that is too soft, masked by ambient noise, or outside the detectable range (perhaps due to high-frequency hearing loss).

✦ *Sample use error:* User does not hear a high-priority alarm indicating that the device is running out of battery power.

✦ *Consequence:* Device might run out of power at an inopportune time, which could lead to harm.

INCONSPICUOUS PLACEMENT

✦ *Problem:* Users can overlook an inconspicuous control or display (including labels).

✦ *Sample use error:* User does not notice a warning about not using an intravenous infusion tubing set to deliver whole blood.

✦ *Consequence:* User might deliver whole blood through a tubing set that causes damage to the blood cells.

INSUFFICIENT TOUCH SCREEN SENSITIVITY

✦ *Problem:* Users are more prone to input errors when a touch screen does not respond reliably to a touch, perhaps due to screen contamination and overly light touches.

✦ *Sample use error:* User intended to program an infusion pump to deliver a medication at a rate of 200 mg/hour and touches the "2," "0," and "0" keys properly, but the touch screen registers only the first "0" and not the second "0."

✦ *Consequence:* Patient receives a medication underdose.

LIMITED DISPLAY VIEWING ANGLE

✦ *Problem:* Users cannot read a display when viewing it from more than a 45° offset angle.

✦ *Sample use error:* User does not unclamp one of the fluid lines as directed by the onscreen instructions because the instructions are not legible from the user's viewing angle.

✦ *Consequence:* Dialysis machine "pulls" more fluid than prescribed from the patient.

MUFFLED SOUND

✦ *Problem:* Users might not detect an alarm or other important acoustic feedback produced by a speaker that becomes muffled by clothing, pillows, or other objects that absorb sound.

✦ *Sample use error:* User does not hear the alarm tone produced by a wearable infusion pump because she is wearing several layers of clothing, including a winter parka that cover the device.

✦ *Consequence:* User does not detect an alarm tone indicating that there is an insulin infusion line blockage, resulting in high blood glucose due to an insulin underdose (Figure 10.2).

NARROW AND SHALLOW HANDLES

✦ *Problem:* Users have difficulty holding a large device because the device's molded handles are narrow and shallow, thereby preventing a secure, multiple-finger grip.

✦ *Sample use error:* User drops a patient monitor while transporting it from one point-of-care setting to another.

✦ *Consequence:* Patient monitor falls on and breaks the user's toe.

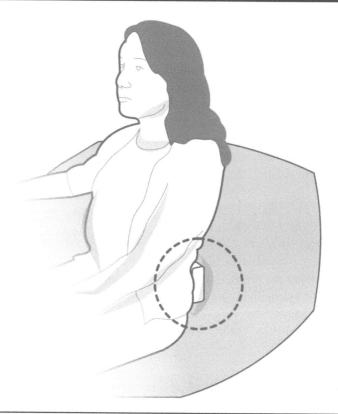

FIGURE 10.2 A device's alarms can be muffled by the surrounding objects, such as seat cushions.

No Functional Grouping

✦ *Problem:* Users can be confused and feel overwhelmed by control panels that have an extensive number of unsegregated controls.

✦ *Sample use error:* A sonographer adjusts the wrong rotary knob on an ultrasound scanner's control panel, thereby setting the wrong depth of energy penetration.

✦ *Consequence:* Ultrasound images have less clarity and lead to an incorrect diagnosis.

No Safeguard

✦ *Problem:* Users can unintentionally activate or deactivate a device function when the control is exposed to inadvertent actuation.

✦ *Sample use error:* User bumps against a device's power button, unintentionally turning it off.

✦ *Consequence:* Patient is deprived of therapy.

No Spotlighting

+ *Problem:* Users might not notice important features when using a device in dim lighting conditions.
+ *Sample use error:* User presses test strip against a blood glucose meter's case rather than guiding it into the test strip port.
+ *Consequence:* Test strip is damaged and it prevents the user from obtaining a blood glucose reading.

No Strain Relief

+ *Problem:* Users can arrange device tubes and cables in a manner that causes them to bend sharply.
+ *Sample use error:* In the process of installing a blood tubing set on a dialysis machine, the user bends a blood tube sharply to route it in the preferred direction.
+ *Consequence:* As the blood tube warms up because of warm blood flowing through it, its sidewalls bend enough to create a partial occlusion (i.e., kink) that leads to hemolysis (damage to the red blood cells) due to high-velocity flow and shearing.

Pinch Point

+ *Problem:* A pinch point, such as might be created by a hospital bed's guardrail when it moves up and down, can cause traumatic injury to a user's body part (e.g., crushing a finger). It might also compress or shear a tube or cable.
+ *Sample use error:* User does not take care to guide an intravenous infusion tube away from the pinch point, and subsequently the tube becomes occluded by the pinching force imparted by a bed's guardrail (when placed in the low position).
+ *Consequence:* Patient does not receive essential drug therapy (e.g., does not receive antibiotic in a timely manner).

Requires Too Much Dexterity

+ *Problem:* Users might not have the physical dexterity to perform certain manual tasks.
+ *Sample use error:* User cannot open a device's battery door to replace its battery.
+ *Consequence:* Device runs out of power (Figure 10.3).

Sharp Edge

+ *Problem:* A sharp edge, such as might be found on a device's enclosure, can cause an abrasion or laceration. It might perforate personal

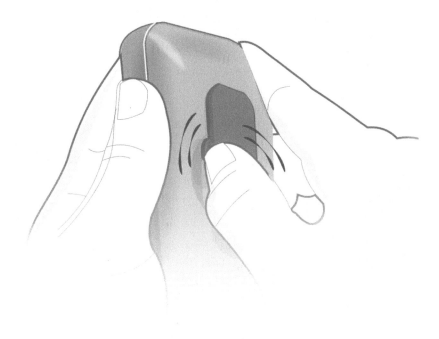

FIGURE 10.3 A user struggles to open a device's battery door because it requires too much dexterity to open.

protective equipment that is intended to prevent exposure to harmful materials (e.g., pathogens, chemicals). A sharp edge might also damage devices that come into contact with it.

✦ *Sample use error:* Repeated rubbing between a sharp edge and a fluid line eventually wears a hole in the line and causes a fluid leak.

✦ *Consequence:* Patient does not receive essential drug therapy (e.g., medication to control blood pressure is not received in a timely manner).

SIMILAR COLORS

✦ *Problem:* Users can confuse similar items that have the same or nearly the same color.

✦ *Sample use error:* Pharmacist erroneously fills a prescription with a higher concentration of the prescribed drug, mistaking the "medium-blue" carton for the "light-blue" carton.

✦ *Consequence:* User receives overdose due to treatment with higher concentration drug.

WIDELY COMPATIBLE CONNECTORS

✦ *Problem:* Users can connect tubes and cables to the wrong ports when visual and tactile cues regarding the proper connections are insufficient and when such connections are physically possible.

✦ *Sample use error:* User connects an oxygen tube (originally intended for connection to a nebulizer) to an intravenous access (e.g., Luer-activated valve).

✦ *Consequence:* High-pressure oxygen flows into the patient's bloodstream.

SOFTWARE USER INTERFACE DESIGN FLAW EXAMPLES

ABBREVIATION

✦ *Problem:* Some users might be unfamiliar with the meaning of a particular abbreviation.

✦ *Sample use error:* User does not recognize the meaning of "EXP" to be "expiration date" and, therefore, does not recognize that a prefilled syringe contains an expired drug.

✦ *Consequence:* User injects an expired drug that might no longer be efficacious.

INFORMATION DENSITY

✦ *Problem:* Users can be overwhelmed by various types of media (e.g., computer display, instruction sheet) that present a lot of information in a limited space, thereby leading them to disregard the information or take more time than expected to find information.

✦ *Sample use error:* User reads only a portion of the instructions on how to operate a nebulizer and, therefore, does not read the instruction to wash the device in a special solution.

✦ *Consequence:* User does not fully disinfect the nebulizer, thereby increasing the chance of inhaling bacteria during the next use.

INSUFFICIENT VISUAL HIERARCHY

✦ *Problem:* Users have difficulty focusing on the most important information first when a screen does not present information in some form of visual hierarchy, which can be based on information labeling, layout, size, color, and dynamic effects (e.g., pulsing).

✦ *Sample use error:* When reviewing a patient record on an electronic health record (EHR), the user does not notice text indicating that

the patient has an allergy to sulfonamides (i.e., sulfa drugs) and prescribes Bactrim (a sulfa drug) to treat an ear infection.

✦ *Consequence:* The patient develops a severe skin rash in reaction to
the drug.

LOW CONTRAST

✦ *Problem:* Low contrast between text and its backgrounds can lead
users to overlook information or make it difficult for users to read the
information correctly or at all.

✦ *Sample use error:* User misreads the infusion rate to be 3.5 rather
than 3.2.

✦ *Consequence:* User stops the infusion in progress to adjust the infusion rate, delaying drug delivery (Figure 10.4).

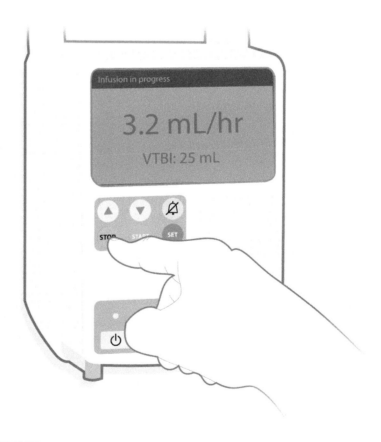

FIGURE 10.4   An infusion pump with low contrast between the screen's text and
background.

No Confirmation

✦ *Problem:* Users might have difficulty detecting a use error and/or correcting it when they are not given the chance to confirm an action before it takes effect.

✦ *Sample use error:* User stops a dialysis machine's blood pump because he inadvertently pressed the wrong touch screen key and was not given the opportunity to cancel the consequential action.

✦ *Consequence:* The blood pump stops, unnecessarily suspending an important therapy. It takes the user several minutes to notice the inadvertent outcome. Blood may start to coagulate in the blood tubing set and dialyzer, thereby posing the risk of a clot entering the patient's bloodstream when the pump restarts, or requiring the time-consuming and costly replacement of the blood tubing set.

No Data Validity Checks

✦ *Problem:* Users are prone to data entry errors and might not catch the errors if a device or application does not have built-in data validity checks.

✦ *Sample use error:* A nurse enters the wrong narcotic drug dose rate into an infusion pump. The dose rate far exceeds the recommended maximum.

✦ *Consequence:* The patient receives an overdose of narcotic.

Poor Information Layout

✦ *Problem:* Users have difficulty acquiring and entering information when screen content layout lacks underlying logic and particularly when the physical layout does not match the natural workflow.

✦ *Sample use error:* A user does not confirm changes to a patient monitor's alarm limits settings. Rather, he changes the settings without pressing the "Done" button and, after a minute passes, the monitor defaults back to the previously set alarm limits.

✦ *Consequence:* The monitor does not alert clinicians to a vital sign (e.g., systolic blood pressure) that is outside the healthy range as described by the intended modified alarm limits.

Small Decimal Point

✦ *Problem:* Users might overlook a particularly small decimal point and misread a number.

✦ *Sample use error:* User reads the number as "27" when it is actually "2.7."

✦ *Consequence:* User might administer the wrong therapy after misreading the parameter value.

SMALL TEXT

✦ *Problem:* Small text can lead users to overlook information or make it difficult for users to read the information correctly.

✦ *Sample use error:* User did not notice that the infusion set was not intended for the intravenous delivery of whole blood.

✦ *Consequence:* In the absence of proper blood filtering, transfused blood contained clots that formed during blood collection and storage, posing the risk of an embolism.

TOGGLE AMBIGUITY

✦ *Problem:* Due to the specific design and labeling of controls (hardware or software based), users might have difficulty determining if actuating a control will produce the intended or opposite effect.

✦ *Sample use error:* Faced with a dark gray button labeled "ON" in white text and a white button labeled "OFF" in black text, the user erroneously presses the white button to turn a function on.

✦ *Consequence:* User does not recognize a function's true status and/or switches the function to the wrong status.

DOCUMENT USER INTERFACE DESIGN FLAW EXAMPLES

BINDING DOES NOT FACILITATE HANDS-FREE USE

✦ *Problem:* Users might need to use both hands to operate a device while simultaneously reading a document. This is problematic when a document will not stay open to a selected page.

✦ *Sample use error:* A user stopped trying to follow a heart pump battery exchange procedure because the user manual's binding kept causing it to close.

✦ *Consequence:* User causes the heart pump to stop briefly due to a power loss because she did not follow the correct battery exchange procedure.

BLACK AND WHITE PRINTING LIMITS COMPREHENSION

✦ *Problem:* The illustrated patient insert uses black and white line drawings to present assembly instructions for a nasal delivery device.

✦ *Sample use error:* User removes incorrect cap and attaches vial to the wrong end of the nasal delivery device because the illustration lacks salient details to distinguish the components.

✦ *Consequence:* User breaks the vial, resulting in no dose delivery.

No Graphical Reinforcement

✦ *Problem:* The lack of graphical illustration can leave users confused about how to perform a task.

✦ *Sample use error:* The user does not recognize where to look for large air bubbles in a syringe.

✦ *Consequence:* User injects drug containing air bubbles into his body. Although the intramuscular injection of a large air bubble is not consequential, the void created by the air bubble in the syringe barrel leads to a drug underdose.

No Index

✦ *Problem:* Users sometimes struggle to find information of interest, or at least to find it quickly, when there is no index to facilitate the search.

✦ *Sample use error:* A dialysis nurse does not find the detailed guidance on how to load a syringe filled with heparin into the machine's built-in syringe pump.

✦ *Consequence:* The syringe flanges are not properly seated in the pump's drive mechanism and, therefore, cause the plunger tip to become displaced from the drive mechanism. This halts the flow of heparin and increases the chance of blood clotting in the dialyzer.

No Troubleshooting Section

✦ *Problem:* Users facing difficulties with device operation frequently seek troubleshooting advice from a user manual, and they might fail to solve a problem or at least take more time to do so if the content is absent.

✦ *Sample use error:* A dialysis technician takes far more time than desirable to eliminate an air bubble in a blood return line.

✦ *Consequence:* The dialysis treatment is delayed and the risk of returning clotted blood to the patient increases.

Poor Information Coding

✦ *Problem:* Lack of distinction between procedural steps and supporting narrative content.

✦ *Sample use error:* The user overlooks the instruction to disinfect a pen-injector's septum before attaching a needle.

✦ *Consequence:* There is an increased chance of the injection causing a bacterial infection if the septum was contaminated.

POOR INFORMATION PLACEMENT

✦ *Problem:* Important information is "buried" in the back of a large document. Therefore, users might be oversaturated with warnings of various importance and not bother to review all of them.

✦ *Sample use error:* A user cannot find troubleshooting information because it is placed in the back of the document along with device technical specifications and away from user-oriented information.

✦ *Consequence:* User cannot resolve difficulty in getting nebulizer treatment to begin.

UNCONVENTIONAL WARNINGS

✦ *Problem:* Warnings do not reflect the conventional prioritization scheme that employs various signal words (e.g., DANGER, WARNING, CAUTION, and NOTICE).

✦ *Sample use error:* A fentanyl drug patch user faced with a page of marginally differentiated text does not read the warning about not drinking alcohol while wearing the patch.

✦ *Consequence:* User experiences severe low blood pressure caused by the interaction effect of the drug and alcohol. (Figure 10.5).

UNFAMILIAR LANGUAGE

✦ *Problem:* Users can experience difficulty understanding documents that are written in unfamiliar technical terms such as those used by engineers or, simply stated, documents that do not "speak their language."

✦ *Sample use error:* A nurse assistant does not understand the Instructions for Use's procedural guidance on how to "pair" a portable patient monitor with data receiver and, therefore, cannot upload monitored parameter values.

✦ *Consequence:* A clinician responsible for remotely monitoring a patient's condition does not receive current data in time to diagnose a worsening condition.

VISUAL INTERFERENCE

✦ *Problem:* Some instruction sheets are so thin that content printed on one side is visible on the other side (i.e., it bleeds through), thereby making the document less readable.

FIGURE 10.5   Documents lacking (left) and containing (right) conventional signal words.

✦ *Sample use error:* User does not comprehend the graphic showing how to properly twist an infusion line onto an insulin pump because the graphic is visually obscured by another graphic and text that is bleeding through from the other side of the instruction sheet.

✦ *Consequence:* User fails to attach the infusion line to the insulin pump properly, causing the infusion line to come loose from the insulin pump, thereby spilling insulin and halting the therapy.

PACKAGING USER INTERFACE DESIGN FLAW EXAMPLES

"HIDDEN" INSTRUCTIONS

✦ *Problem:* Users do not find the Instructions for Use because they are placed in an inconspicuous sleeve within the associated device's carton.

✦ *Sample use error:* User does not wash a brand new nebulizer's components prior to use.

✦ *Consequence:* User inhales fine particles remaining on the device as a consequence of the manufacturing and packaging process (Figure 10.6).

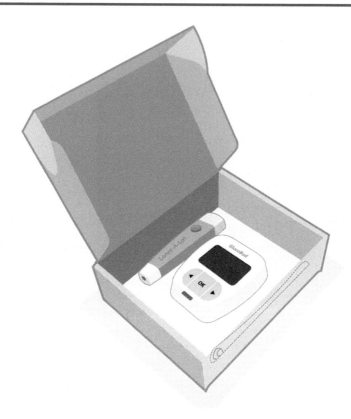

FIGURE 10.6 Example of an Instructions for Use document rolled up and "hidden" in a package containing a glucose meter and lancing device.

INCONSPICUOUS AND DIFFICULT-TO-READ EXPIRATION DATE

✦ *Problem:* Users can fail to notice an expiration date printed in small text embedded with secondary text on the back of the package, where it is less likely to be noticed.

✦ *Sample use error:* The user loads an auto-injector with an expired cartridge due to overlooking the expiration date on the cartridge's package.

✦ *Consequence:* User injects degraded drug that is less potent, leading to an underdose.

LIMITED FINGER ACCESS

✦ *Problem:* Users have difficulty removing components from a package without damaging them because there is poor finger access into the containment slot.

✦ *Sample use error:* User bends a portion of a catheter while removing it from its package.

✦ *Consequence:* Catheter components require more force to advance and retract them, changing the device's "feel."

SHARP EDGE

✦ *Problem:* Package has a sharp edge, compounded by the absence of a visually obvious instruction on how to open the package.

✦ *Sample use error:* User tries tearing open the relatively thick plastic package, loses her grip, and swipes her hand against the package's sharp edge.

✦ *Consequence:* User suffers a minor laceration.

SMALL TEXT

✦ *Problem:* Users might not notice the difference between two packages that contain different doses (e.g., 100 mg and 200 mg) of the same medication.

✦ *Sample use error:* Pharmacist selects the wrong carton of medication from a pharmacy shelf.

✦ *Consequence:* Patient obtains the incorrect medication and receives either an underdose or overdose.

For additional examples of use errors and root causes, as well as suggested mitigations for addressing user interface design flaws, see Chapter 12.

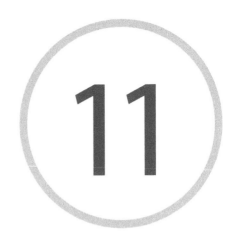

Reporting Root Causes of Medical Device Use Error

INTRODUCTION

In Chapter 12, we describe root causes of many different types of use errors. Such root causes are usually reported to regulatory authorities (FDA in particular) in a broader context that includes the following elements:

+ Succinct title describing the error.
+ Risk identifier—a cross reference to the risk analysis (e.g., failure modes and effects analysis) line item related to the use error.
+ Risk priority number, and possibly the use error's likelihood and the severity ratings from which it is derived.
+ Potential harms that result from the use error, which may be extracted from the risk analysis. Note that some regulators have

requested detailed descriptions of harms (e.g., a paragraph instead of a sentence or phrase).

✦ Usability test task during which the use error occurred.

✦ Task priority (e.g., priority 1 of 10) among all tasks performed during the usability test.

✦ Use error occurrences, which may be expressed as a total number of use errors, a use error rate, and in some cases as a percentage of how many test participants committed the use error.

✦ Identifiers of participants who committed the use error (e.g., the first patient participant is identified as P1 and the first healthcare professional participant is identified as HCP1).

✦ Detailed use error description.

✦ Participant-reported root causes.

✦ Root cause analysis, including a brief title and description of each root cause.

✦ Residual risk analysis, which may indicate the need for further risk control or suggest that the risk is reasonably low, so there is no need for further risk control.

In the following text, we present a couple of hypothetical use error reports that include the elements listed previously, noting that other formats containing the same elements would be fine. In these examples, we focus on reporting use errors, but the same general format would apply in your reports of close calls, operational difficulties, and instances of test administrator assistance.

DID NOT ATTACH NEEDLE SECURELY

RISK IDENTIFIER

- Report: ACME-FMEA-WIDGET-134627.Rev1
- Line item: 16.3, incomplete needle attachment
- Risk priority number: 15: likelihood = 5, severity = 3

POTENTIAL HARMS

- Underdose due to fluid leaking out of pen-injector at injector–needle connection.
- Systemic infection due to reuse of contaminated needle (if needle falls off pen-injector and user puts it back on).
- Additional pain due to need to perform a second injection to deliver full dose.

TASKS

- 6—Deliver 20 units of insulin
- 7—Deliver 10 units of insulin

Task priorities: Task 6: 4 of 8, Task 7: 5 of 8

OCCURRENCES

Five out of 30 participants committed this use error one or more times during five repeated injection trials. The use error occurred five times out of the 60 opportunities to err, yielding a use error rate of 8.3%.

(Test participant identifiers: P1, P5, P18, P29, P30)

DESCRIPTION

Three participants (P5, P18, P30) pressed the needle onto the pen-injector but did not twist the needle to lock it in place.

Two participants (P1, P29) initially twisted the needle to lock it in place, but then unlocked it when they removed the needle cap by means of a twisting, rather than pulling, motion.

PARTICIPANT-REPORTED ROOT CAUSES

Three participants (P5, P18, P30) said they forgot to twist the needle to lock it in place.

Two participants (P1, P29) speculated that they must have initially gripped the needle's hub, rather than the cap, when removing the needle cap, thereby loosening the needle.

ROOT CAUSE ANALYSIS

- *Locked needle not distinguishable.* There is no visual feedback to distinguish a needle that is locked in place from one that is not. (P1, P5, P18, P29, P30)
- *Needle cap gripping surface close to needle hub.* The needle cap gripping surface is adjacent to the needle hub, making the needle hub vulnerable to unintended twisting during cap removal. (P1, P29)

RESIDUAL RISK ANALYSIS (APPEARING IN ACME'S HFE REPORT)

There is no need for additional risk control.

ACME considers the residual risk associated with not attaching the needle securely to the pen-injector to be reasonably low and that there is no need for additional risk control. Specific rationales follow:

- The potential underdose due to fluid leaking out of the pen-injector at the injector–needle connection is likely to be small (≤1 unit of insulin). Also, the user is likely to notice the leaking fluid and take future precautions to avoid such leakage by attaching the needle securely, noting that four out of five participants noticed leaking fluid. Therefore, ACME does not expect users to repeat this use error, recognizing that none of the test participants committed the use error more than once despite having the opportunity to do so during subsequent tasks.

- The potential harm due to re-using the contaminated needle (if the needle falls off the pen-injector and the user puts it back on) is that the user will develop an infection at the injection site. Such an infection is likely to be minor. The user's immune system is likely to fight the infection effectively, with or without the administration of antibiotics.

- The additional pain due to the need to perform a second injection to deliver a full dose is likely to be minor. The ultra-fine needle (31 gauge) causes little if any pain. Moreover, users are accustomed to delivering several injections each day and an extra needle stick is unlikely to be a cause for concern.

SIDEBAR 11.1   ASSIGNING ROOT CAUSES TO PARTICIPANTS

When reporting root causes, you should assign root causes to participants (i.e., identify the one or more participants to whom each root cause applies). Most often, there is more than one root cause associated with a given use error. For example, a participant might enter a value incorrectly and fail to notice her mistake due in part to the numeric keypad's small size. However, you might also identify the lack of a confirmation screen as a contributing root cause. As such, when you are reporting root causes, it is important to consider that you can attribute a single participant's use error to more than one root cause. Moreover, participants themselves might report multiple root causes for a single use error.

Additionally, when several participants commit the same use error, it is possible that the full set of root causes you identified in the course of completing your analysis might not apply to each participant. As an example, three participants might commit the same use error, such as setting an incorrect dose. You might attribute two of these participants' use errors to the dose display's small text, which led the participants to misread the dose. Then, you might attribute the third participant's use error to habit, because the participant intentionally selected the dose he administers at home, rather than the dose listed in the task prescription card. In these situations, the use error report's root cause analysis section should specify to which participants each root cause applies.

We suggest listing the root causes in order of frequency (i.e., list the root cause assigned to the most participants first, followed by root causes assigned to fewer participants). This approach typically results in presenting the root cause that has the largest role in causing the use error first, followed by root causes that had less impact. If there are no differences in frequency (i.e., each root cause is assigned to the same number of participants), we recommend listing design-related root causes first, followed by other types of root causes (e.g., test artifact, habit).

DID NOT IDENTIFY THAT PATIENT ADMINISTERED A PARTIAL DOSE

RISK IDENTIFIER(S)

- Report: ACME-FMEA-WIDGET-134627.Rev1
- Line item: 30.1, HCP misinterpreted medication adherence
- Risk priority number: 12: likelihood = 4, severity = 3

POTENTIAL HARM

- Repeated medication underdose

TASK

- 2—Interpret medication adherence

Task priority: 2 of 8

OCCURRENCES

One out of 18 participants committed this use error one time. The use error occurred one time out of the 36 opportunities to err, yielding a use error rate of 2.8%.
(Test participant identifier: HCP9)

DESCRIPTION

One participant (HCP9) did not identify that the patient administered a partial (i.e., incomplete) dose of medication on January 2. Instead, the participant reported that the patient administered all doses correctly in January.

PARTICIPANT-REPORTED ROOT CAUSE

The participant reported that he did not realize the patient administered a partial dose on January 2 because the partial dose indicator looks very similar to the complete dose indicator on the "Monthly Medication Adherence" screen.

ROOT CAUSE ANALYSIS

- *Partial dose indicator not distinguished.* The "Monthly Medication Adherence" screen indicates days with complete doses and partial doses by using filled and partially filled dark blue squares, respectively. The filled and partially filled squares look nearly identical. As such, the participant mistook the partially filled square for a filled square (i.e., he concluded incorrectly that the partial dose was a complete dose). This led him to conclude incorrectly that the patient administered a complete dose on January 2. (HCP9)

RESIDUAL RISK ANALYSIS (APPEARING IN ACME'S HFE REPORT): ADDITIONAL RISK CONTROL REQUIRED

ACME considers the residual risk associated with misinterpreting the medication adherence information to be unacceptable. As such, ACME will implement additional risk control measures to reduce the risk further.

Note: This form of use error report would not appear in an HFE report to the FDA or other regulator because the manufacturer has decided that a design modification is warranted. After the manufacturer implements the modification, it should update the residual risk analysis to include a description of the modification and the results on the remaining residual risk analysis (presumably, that the residual risk is reasonably low and that there is no need for additional risk control).

DISTINGUISHING FACTS AND HYPOTHESES

When reporting root causes, it is important to distinguish between facts and hypotheses. Suppose you tested a dialysis machine that requires patients to open or break a seal (i.e., peel seam) between two compartments of dialysate to mix them properly before use (Figure 11.1).

Now, suppose that one test participant could not break the seal between the two fluid compartments and during a post-task interview stated:

Anecdotal comment: "I couldn't get the two fluids to mix no matter how hard I tried to squeeze and press on the two compartments."

In this case, you could confidently report this finding as a fact:

Fact: "The participant reported that breaking the seal between the two fluid compartments required more force than he could exert."

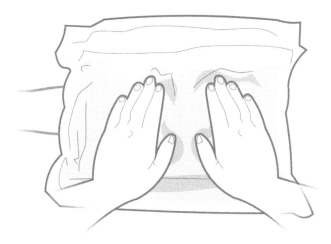

FIGURE 11.1   Dialysate bag with two compartments.

Your root cause analysis could be equally definitive:

Fact: "Breaking the seal between the two fluid compartments required more force than the participant could exert when squeezing the compartments or pressing on them with the bag placed on a countertop."

Next, suppose that one test participant did not notice that the bag of dialysate was past its expiration date and during a post-task interview stated:

Anecdotal comment: "I guess I forgot to check the expiration date. But it doesn't really stand out much, so it is easy to forget. I can read it just fine, but it looks unimportant compared to other information."

In this case, you can report the test participant's comment factually:

Fact: "The participant reported that he forgot to read the expiration date."

However, your root cause analysis should be worded as a hypothesis rather than a fact:

Hypothesis: "The expiration date, which is printed in small (10-point) text, *does not seem* sufficiently conspicuous to ensure that users notice it and perform the necessary step to check it.

The reason to hypothesize by using the expression "does not seem" is that larger text might or might not draw more attention or serve as a helpful reminder to check the expiration date. You would need to conduct a study to prove the benefit of large text and such a study would likely be outside the scope of the root cause analysis. Therefore, although larger text is likely to reduce the chance of the cited use error, the small text remains a hypothetical root cause of the reported use error.

Ultimately, hypothesizing is really about hedging—recognizing that you are making a judgment call rather than stating a fact.

RESIDUAL RISK ANALYSIS

Although this book is about root cause analysis of use error and not specifically about the topic of residual risk analysis, here is some advice about the kind of content to include in the residual risk analysis section of your use error report.

+ **Outcome of residual risk analysis.** State the outcome of your residual risk analysis. For example, if you determined that the residual risk is reasonably low, indicate this result, noting that no further risk controls are necessary. Alternatively, if the residual risk remains unacceptably high, then indicate that further risk mitigations are warranted.

✦ **Test participant comments.** The residual risk analysis may be reinforced by test participant comments, including those pertaining to detecting problems, which suggest that people are less likely to repeat the use error and/or intervene before the error causes significant harm.

✦ **Results of medical studies.** The residual risk analysis may include much more detail than shown in the preceding examples. Companies may choose to present an expanded medical explanation of the level of harm that might be caused by the cited use error, or provide a cross reference to another study that discusses the potential harm. As mentioned before, some regulators are seeking more detailed descriptions of harm so that they can better understand the consequences of a given use error.

✦ **Description of existing safety features.** Take credit for user interface features that you consider to be safety features. You might have added these features in response to earlier study findings, suggesting that you have enhanced the design as much as possible.

PRESENTING THE RESULTS OF A RESIDUAL RISK ANALYSIS

Use errors observed during a summative usability test are typically documented in two places: (1) the summative usability test report and (2) the final HFE report submitted to FDA and possibly other regulatory authorities. A summative usability test report describes the results of the usability test, whereas an HFE report (per FDA's guidance[*]) summarizes many of the HFE activities performed throughout the product's development, and particularly the results of the summative usability test.

After completing a summative usability test, those who conducted the summative test (e.g., HFE consultants, internal HFE team) document all use errors in the summative usability test report. The test report should include all the reporting elements described earlier, with the exception of the residual risk analysis. Companies must first consider the use errors observed during the summative test (i.e., the results documented in the summative test report), and then proceed to perform the residual risk analysis. As such, the results of the residual risk analysis are not typically presented in the

---

[*] "FDA's Draft Guidance for Industry and Food and Drug Administration Staff—Applying Human Factors and Usability Engineering to Optimize Medical Device Design" (issued June 22, 2011).

stand-alone test report, particularly if the test report is written for a company by a consultant. That said, it would be more appropriate, but not necessary in view of the HFE report's contents, for test reports generated by in-house test teams to include residual risk analysis. If a company is not submitting a device for clearance by FDA, residual risk analysis results may be added to the summative usability test report.

Companies often take a similar reporting approach when dealing with adverse events. The initial adverse event report details the event, including information such as a description of the event and the date on which the event occurred. Then, a follow-up report describes the outcome of the residual risk analysis.

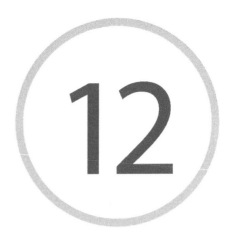

Root Cause Analysis Examples

ABOUT THE ROOT CAUSE ANALYSIS EXAMPLES

This chapter illustrates use errors resulting from user interface shortcomings and shows design modifications that might help in preventing such errors. Our illustrative format is different from the more "cut and dried" one used to report root cause analysis in a usability test report or adverse event report (see Chapter 11). Here, we have taken a more visual approach that cites potential solutions to user interface design flaws, with the goal of making the book more helpful to readers who would like to read about solutions in addition to problems.

Regulators do not necessarily expect root cause analysis discussions in a summative usability test report—or an adverse event report, for that matter—to be as richly illustrated as presented in these examples. That said, an informative drawing or photo can be a helpful complement to a narrative discussion.

Each of the 30 examples in this chapter includes the following contents:

+ Product description
+ Use error title

- Use error description, including participants' speculations (i.e., subjective feedback) regarding the use error's root cause, written in a conversational manner
- Potential harms resulting from the use error, matching those listed in a use-related failure modes and effects analysis (or equivalent risk analysis form)
- Root cause(s) with concise rationales
- Suggested mitigations

Our hope is that these examples educate readers on a wide variety of potential root causes of medical device use errors. Many of the root causes describe common flaws we see in medical devices, but we also explore other types of root causes, including test artifact, user's habits, and negative transfer. The examples cover a wide range of medical devices, including home-use products such as a nebulizer, pen-injector, and smartphone applications, as well as devices used in clinical environments, such as a blood gas analyzer, a ventricular assist device, and an ultrasound machine.

A few more things you should know about the examples include

- We begin each example with a product description to give readers a sense for the device's function, intended users, and use environment. However, this information is not normally included within individual use error reports.
- The use errors are hypothetical but inspired, at least in some cases, by shortcomings in actual products that we have observed or read about.
- Although also hypothetical, the sample participant comments about the use errors typify those that we hear during interviews with test participants and people who have committed errors using medical devices to deliver actual care. As such, the comments purposefully sound informal, vary in their level of detail, and do not always identify the correct root cause of the cited use error.
- We present sample harms that can result from each use error. We based these listed harms on our research, experience, and judgment. In a real root cause analysis, you should defer to medical experts to define harms.
- You might disagree with our root cause analyses and suggested mitigations, noting that they reflect the kinds of judgments that we discussed in Chapter 2.
- The suggested mitigations are based on human factors engineering design principles, but we acknowledge that they might or might not be effective. The effectiveness of any design mitigation can be

determined only by having representative users interact with the modified device and seeing if they perform tasks correctly or if they still make mistakes.

✦ We present a few sample mitigations for each use error, but the list is not comprehensive, recognizing that there is often more than one design change that can address the use error. As such, readers might have other, equally valid ideas for opportunities to mitigate against a given use error.

✦ The examples cover a wide range of medical devices, but stop short of including highly advanced systems that might require coordination among multiple users or involve the use of multiple devices. Root cause analyses of such advanced systems require detail beyond describing a particular device and the comments that a user might make about a particular use error. For the sake of keeping the examples clear and concise, we omitted such advanced systems from this chapter.

✦ In an actual usability test report or adverse event report, root cause rationales may be more expansive, given that the report's primary purpose is to fully inform the reader (e.g., a regulatory official reviewing the report)—a goal that might require more than a paragraph or two. Chapter 11 presents two examples of how you can report use errors and root causes in a summative usability report. You will see that they are indeed more "cut and dried."

✦ Root cause analysis may also be informed by analytical end-products, such as an Ishikawa (i.e., fishbone) diagram or AcciMap, for example (see Chapter 14). These products are not normally included in a usability test or adverse event reports, although they may be included in a human factors design history file.

We thank our colleague and this book's illustrator—Jonathan Kendler—for the fine visual explanations that enrich the root cause analysis examples. Indeed, each illustration saved us from writing and you from having to read a thousand more words (conciseness is a virtue). In fact, we took the same advice offered in the form of a suggested mitigation in the example of the ultrasonic nebulizer: augment written instructions with graphics.

Product

Insulin Pen-Injector

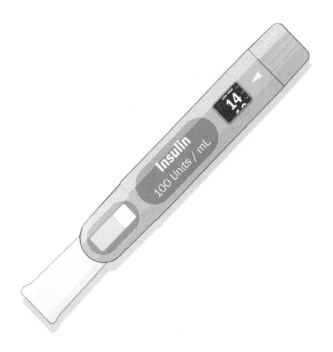

FIGURE 12.1   An insulin pen-injector.

An insulin pen-injector enables people who have diabetes to inject various forms of insulin to help control their blood sugar level (Figure 12.1). They may use the device at home and in other environments, including in their cars, workplaces, restaurants, theaters, and outdoor settings. Some users might have diabetes-related impairments, such as numb fingertips (due to peripheral neuropathy) and blurred or black-spotted vision (due to retinopathy).

Use Error

SET INCORRECT DOSE

The participant set (i.e., dialed) a dose of 13 units of insulin instead of the prescribed 12 units. He reported, "I felt certain that I set the dose correctly to 12 units. I even double-checked it." Later, he also noted that he could "wiggle" the pen-injector's dose selector and that it did not precisely hold its position at the selected dose. The participant set the dose while viewing the dose window from below; this provided him with a view of the pointer aligning more closely with "12" than "13," which was the actual and incorrect setting (Figure 12.2).

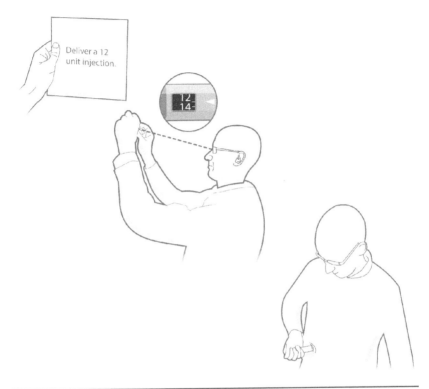

FIGURE 12.2   The task prompt instructed the participant to deliver 12 units of insulin. However, the participant dialed and simulated delivering a dose of 13 units.

Potential harms
+ Mild hypoglycemia

Root Cause #1
PARALLAX

The pen-injector's dose window has a raised plastic frame with a printed, white pointer. As such, the pointer is raised approximately 1.5 mm above the underlying dose indicator. The pointer aligns properly with the intended dose when viewed orthogonally at a 90° angle. However, the pointer becomes visually misaligned when viewed at a sharp angle. Due to parallax,* the pointer

---

* *Parallax* is a condition in which the position or direction of an object appears to differ when viewed from different positions or angles.

can appear to align more closely with the previous or next value on the dose indicator than with the intended one when viewed orthogonally (Figure 12.3).

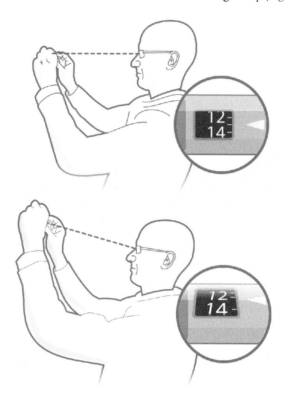

FIGURE 12.3 The set dose can erroneously appear to be "13" rather than the intended "12" when viewed at an angle (from below). The dose of 13 is indicated by the tick mark between doses of 12 and 14.

Root Cause #2
DOSE SELECTOR IMPRECISION

The pen-injector's dose selector does not lock into a precise, unvarying position. Rather, its position relative to the pointer can vary by approximately 50% of the distance between graduations. In other words, the selector has a relatively large amount of "wiggle room" or "backlash" that can exacerbate the parallax problem of misalignment of the pointer and dose setting (Figure 12.4).

Suggested Mitigations
REDESIGN DOSE WINDOW

Redesign the dose window so that the pointer is essentially flush with the numbers on the dose indicator (Figure 12.5).

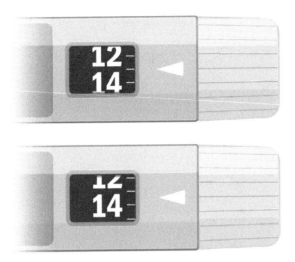

FIGURE 12.4   Due to "wiggle room" in the dose selector, the pointer may not precisely indicate a setting of "13."

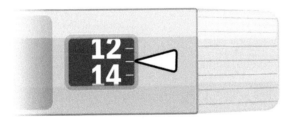

FIGURE 12.5   A revised dose window design with a larger arrow pointer.

REDESIGN DOSE SELECTOR MECHANISM

Redesign the dose selector mechanism so that it stops on and points precisely to each of the individual dose values.

REDESIGN DISPLAY TYPE

Use a display type that is not susceptible to parallax (e.g., a digital display).

Product

Drug Bottle

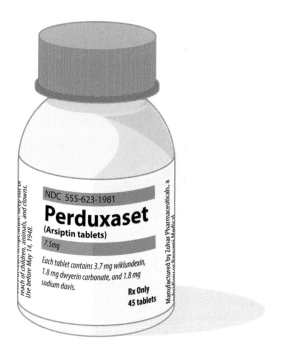

NDC 555-623-1981

Perduxaset

(Arsiptin tablets)

7.5mg

Each tablet contains 3.7 mg wiklundexin, 1.8 mg dwyerin carbonate, and 1.8 mg sodium davis.

Rx Only
45 tablets

FIGURE 12.6   A drug bottle.

The hypothetical drug Perduxaset is a pain medication that comes in three dose strengths (2.5 mg, 5 mg, and 7.5 mg) (Figure 12.6). Pharmacists and pharmacy technicians dispense Perduxaset in retail and hospital pharmacies. These users must select the correct drug (Perduxaset) and dose strength among hundreds of different drugs, all of which are stored on shelving in the pharmacy.

Use Error

SELECTED WRONG DRUG CONCENTRATION

Three pharmacists selected a 7.5 mg strength bottle of Perduxaset instead of a 2.5 mg strength bottle. One participant commented that she had been careless and that she alone was to blame for the mistake. One participant said that he was looking for a bottle of Perduxaset that had a green band on the label and "grabbed" the first one he saw. One participant said she thought the label read 2.5 mg as she reached for the bottle on the highest shelf and did not check it after retrieving it (Figure 12.7).

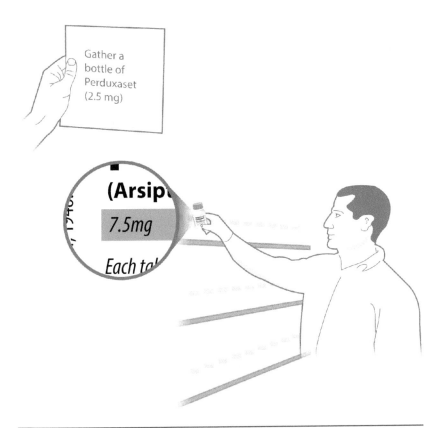

FIGURE 12.7   The participant's task was to gather a 2.5 mg strength bottle of Perduxaset, but he selected the 7.5 mg bottle.

Possible harms

✦   Patient medication overdose

Root Cause #1

INSUFFICIENT CONCENTRATION LABEL DIFFERENTIATION

The Perduxaset concentration labels present black text on green labels that vary only slightly in shade (7.5 mg = medium-dark green, 5 mg = medium green, and 2.5 mg = medium-light green), reportedly to associate color darkness versus lightness with higher versus lower drug concentrations (Figure 12.8).

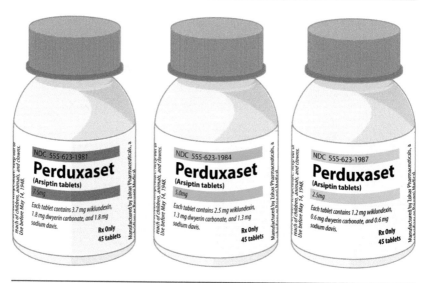

FIGURE 12.8   The three bottles' concentration labels look relatively similar.

Root Cause #2

ILLEGIBLE TEXT

The drug concentration label's legibility is compromised by the use of relatively small (8-point font) numbers and letters. When viewed at a distance of 24 inches, numerals of this size subtend a visual angle of 15.5 arc minutes, which is at the threshold of the recommended visual angle of 16 arc minutes necessary to achieve marginally acceptable legibility.[*]

Root Cause #3

POOR CONTRAST BETWEEN DRUG CONCENTRATION AND BACKGROUND

There is a relatively low contrast ratio between the 7.5 mg bottle label's black characters and the medium-dark green background. Specifically, the label and background have an estimated contrast ratio of 4:1, whereas contrast affording good legibility is in the range of 5:1 to 7:1 or better.[†]

---

[*] ANSI/AAMI HE75:2009/(R)2013, Section 6.2.2.5, "Visual Angle." The standard indicates that the minimum marginally acceptable visual angle is 16 arc minutes.

[†] According to the World Wide Web Consortium's Web "Content Accessibility Guidelines 2.0," a contrast ratio of at least 5:1 to 7:1 will ensure good legibility of text. Available at http://www.w3.org/TR/WCAG20/

Suggested Mitigations

INCREASE NUMBER AND LETTER SIZE

Make the text larger, such as to 18-point font, to increase the drug concentration's legibility.

USE DIFFERENT COLORS TO INDICATE CONCENTRATION

Differentiate multiple concentrations of the same drug using distinctly different color bands that contrast well with either white or black text (Figure 12.9).

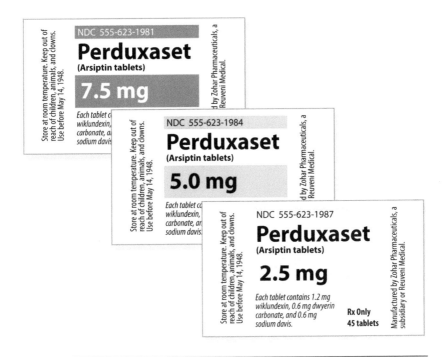

FIGURE 12.9   The revised labels include distinctly different colors and larger text.

Product

Automated External Defibrillator (AED)

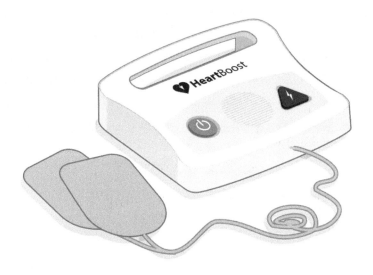

FIGURE 12.10   An automated external defibrillator (AED).

An automated external defibrillator (AED) is a portable device that delivers a cardioverting electric shock to the heart in an attempt to restore a normal sinus rhythm (Figure 12.10). Many AEDs also provide guidance on how to perform effective cardiopulmonary resuscitation (CPR). The devices are present in some homes, but are more commonly found in public settings such as airports, schools, and offices. Intended users include adolescents and adults who can respond effectively to recorded verbal commands and take proper precautions (e.g., do not touch the patient during shock delivery).

Use Error

TOUCHED PATIENT DURING SHOCK DELIVERY

One participant (layperson) touched the simulated patient at the moment the AED delivered a simulated shock. The caregiver's knee contacted the simulated patient's hand, which was stretched out at an approximately 45° angle to the body. The participant explained that she was not particularly concerned about avoiding contact with the simulated patient during the delivery of a simulated shock.

Potential harms
+ Electrical shock

Root Cause #1
LACK OF VOICE COMMAND CLARITY

At the moment preceding shock delivery, the AED emits the voice command, "Stay clear!" This somewhat vague command appears to lack the specificity necessary to compel users, especially non-healthcare professionals, to avoid contact with the patient (Figure 12.11).

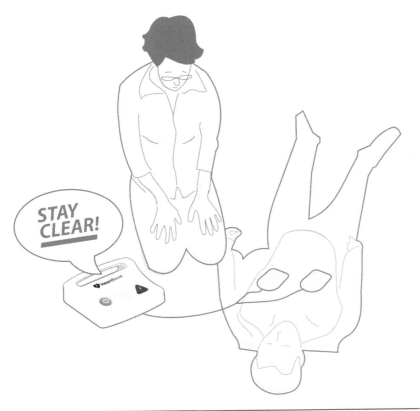

FIGURE 12.11   The "Stay clear!" command did not compel the participant to move her knee away from the patient.

Root Cause #2

TEST ARTIFACT

The test required the participant to simulate administering a treatment (i.e., shock) to a simulated patient a mannequin. The test administrator had previously explained that the participant could not be harmed during the usability test session. The fact that both the shock and the patient were simulated might have compromised the test participant's sense of risk such that she took fewer precautions than she might have taken in a real use scenario.

Suggested Mitigation

REVISE VOICE COMMAND

Revise the voice command to more specifically direct AED users not to touch the patient during shock delivery, for example: "Do not touch the patient."

Product

Handheld Tonometer

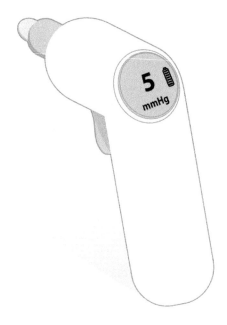

FIGURE 12.12   A handheld tonometer.

A tonometer measures the intraocular pressure (fluid pressure) in the eye's anterior chamber by means of applanation (tapping lightly on the cornea) with a probe connected to a pressure sensor (Figure 12.12). The intended users include eye care professionals (e.g., ophthalmologists and optometrists), who will use the device to screen patients for diseases such as glaucoma. Patients who are at risk for eye problems may also use the device to monitor their eye health. Common tasks include installing a new probe, activating the device, placing the device in the correct position relative to the eye, activating the probe, reading the test result on an embedded display, disposing of the used probe, and deactivating the device.

Use Error

DID NOT COMPLETE FIVE VALID MEASUREMENTS

One participant did not complete the five valid measurements (i.e., eye taps) that enable the device to provide an average intraocular pressure (IOP) value.

Rather, he performed only one valid measurement, as indicated by a single beep, and presumed that he had completed the measurement process. After about 30 seconds, the device timed out and turned off. The participant took the initiative to repeat the task in exactly the same manner, leading to the same result. He concluded that the device was malfunctioning and that he could not complete the task.

Potential harm

✦ Delay in diagnosis of various eye conditions including glaucoma

Root Cause #1

RELIANCE ON USER TO KNOW TO COMPLETE FIVE MEASUREMENTS

The device does not indicate the need to complete five valid measurements before it can calculate and then display an average IOP value. Rather, the device relies on the user to intuit this step (Figure 12.13).

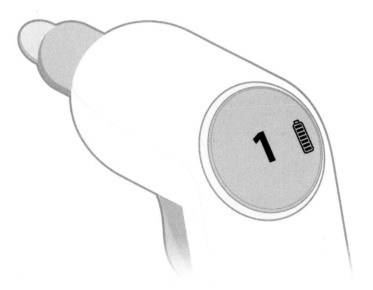

FIGURE 12.13 The display indicates one reading has been completed, but does not prompt the user to perform four more readings.

Root Cause #2

LACK OF FEEDBACK

When the user does not collect five valid IOP measurements within a 30-second period of time, the device times out and turns off. It does not provide the user with any indication that the time available to complete the measurements expired or that five valid IOP measurements were required but not collected.

Suggested Mitigations

ADD PROMPT

Initially display a prompt such as "Measure 5 times in 30 seconds" (Figure 12.14).

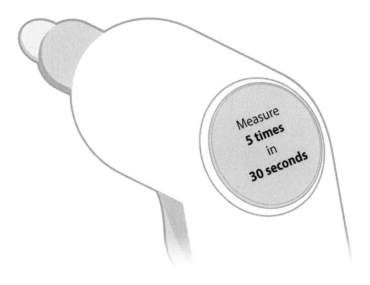

FIGURE 12.14   The revised screen presents an instructional prompt before the user collects the first measurement.

ADD FEEDBACK

Track progress by displaying a message such as "1 of 5 valid IOP measurements." Also, alert the user as the time nears the 30-second expiration and, in the event that the user does not complete five valid measurements within 30 seconds, display a message such as "Time expired. Perform 5 valid IOP measurements within 30 seconds" (Figure 12.15).

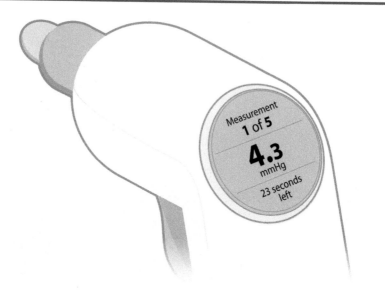

FIGURE 12.15 The revised screen indicates the number of measurements completed and the time remaining to perform additional measurements.

Product
Lancing Device

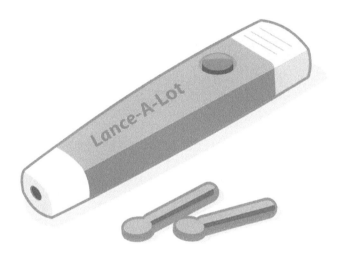

FIGURE 12.16   A lancing device.

A lancing device enables people to "pin prick" their skin to produce a blood droplet (Figure 12.16). Lancing devices are a common part of a blood glucose test kit that also includes test strips and a glucose meter. Users place a lancet (needle) in the lancing device, preload (cock) the lancing device, place its tip over a body part (e.g., fingertip, fleshy portion of forearm), and trigger the device to pierce the underlying skin. After producing a blood droplet, users will touch it to a test strip that is already inserted in a glucose meter. Users range widely in age, including older children, adolescents, adults, and seniors. Individuals could have a wide array of physical impairments, including low vision, hearing loss, and arthritis. Common use environments are the home and workplace, but can include many more settings.

Use Error
REUSED LANCET

One participant drew blood from her fingertip with a lancet that she had previously used, rather than using a new lancet. She commented, "I saw no reason to change the lancet. At home, I use one a half dozen times before discarding it. It saves money. I've never had a problem."

Potential harms
- ✦ Infection
- ✦ Pain (due to dull lancet)

Root Cause #1
WARNING DOES NOT STATE CONSEQUENCE

The lancing device's Instructions for Use (IFU) include a warning directing the user to always use a new lancet. However, this warning does not state the consequence of drawing blood with a used lancet. As such, some users might not recognize the potential harm associated with reusing lancets and, therefore, proceed to reuse one (Figure 12.17).

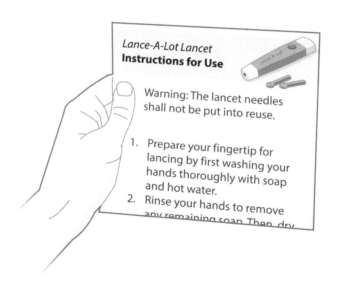

FIGURE 12.17   The IFU's warning message does not state the consequence of reusing a lancet.

Root Cause #2
HABIT

The participant reported that she routinely uses a lancet several times before replacing it. As such, she took the same approach when using this lancing device as a matter of well-established habit.

Suggested Mitigations
EMPHASIZE CONSEQUENCES

Add a statement of consequence to the IFU warning, explaining that reusing lancets can cause pain and possibly lead to infection (Figure 12.18).

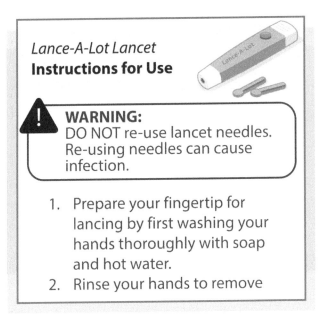

Lance-A-Lot Lancet
Instructions for Use

⚠ **WARNING:**
DO NOT re-use lancet needles. Re-using needles can cause infection.

1. Prepare your fingertip for lancing by first washing your hands thoroughly with soap and hot water.
2. Rinse your hands to remove

FIGURE 12.18   The revised warning message draws attention to the conse-quences associated with reusing a lancet.

PREVENT REUSE

Design the lancing device and/or lancets so that the lancets can be used only once.

Product

Transdermal Patch

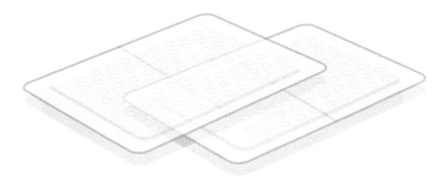

FIGURE 12.19   Two transdermal patches.

A transdermal patch is a medicated adhesive patch that is placed on the skin to deliver a specific dose of a drug through the skin and eventually into the bloodstream (Figure 12.19). Common patch locations include the upper arm, shoulder, back, and thigh. The primary intended users are laypersons. However, healthcare professionals (e.g., nurses) might also be users because they might apply a patch to a patient. User tasks include selecting a fresh patch that has not passed its expiry date, removing the adhesive liner (perhaps in stages if there is more than one), applying the patch to the skin, monitoring the patch area for signs of skin irritation, and removing/replacing the patch at the prescribed interval (e.g., once per day).

Use Error

DID NOT REMOVE BOTH ADHESIVE LINERS

One participant did not remove both adhesive liners from the patch's medicated side before applying the transdermal patch to the simulated skin pad on his abdomen. Rather, he removed only one of the two clear liners. He commented that he would probably use first aid tape to help hold the patch in place, given that the patch did not seem to stick to the simulated skin on one side (the side with the liner still in place).

Later on, during post-task discussions about the use error, the participant said, "I thought I only had to remove a single liner. I didn't notice a second one, but then again I guess I didn't look that closely. The liners are kind of difficult to see because they are clear."

Potential harm
✦ Medication underdose

Root Cause #1
TWO-PIECE LINER

The liner covering the patch's adhesive surface relies on users to recognize that there are two pieces that must be removed. A user who notices only one of the liner's pull-tabs and does not notice the thin demarcation feature (i.e., gap) between the liners might remove only one liner. In lieu of closely inspecting the adhesive surface, the user might conclude that the entire liner has been removed (Figure 12.20).

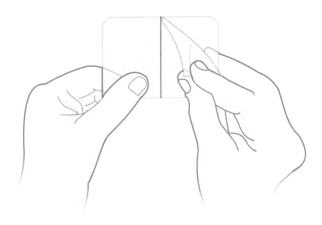

FIGURE 12.20   The user must recognize and remove both liner pieces.

Root Cause #2
CLEAR LINER

The clear liner material and absence of any additional labeling make it relatively difficult to detect that the liner has two pieces. Moreover, it makes it somewhat difficult to distinguish portions of the adhesive pad that are exposed versus remaining covered by the liner.

Root Cause #3
PULL-TAB NOT VISIBLE

The liner's pull-tab rests underneath the patch if the patch is partially applied. As such, the pull-tab portion of a remaining liner piece is not readily visible with the patch pressed against the skin.

Suggested Mitigations
MAKE THE LINER A SINGLE PIECE

Make the liner a single piece so that there is no potential for users to remove only half of it. Design the liner such that users can pull it away partially to position the patch on the skin, and then remove it completely to enable full skin adherence. Ensure that the single-piece liner is not prone to tearing and that the removal action does not cause the adhesive patch to wrinkle or fold onto itself.

COLOR AND LABEL THE LINER

Make the liner opaque (e.g., opaque blue) and add text and/or a graphic instructing the user to remove it before applying the patch to the skin (Figure 12.21).

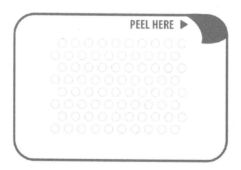

FIGURE 12.21   The revised liner is opaque and includes a "PEEL HERE" label.

EXTEND THE PULL-TABS

Extend the pull-tabs so that they are visible beyond the edge of the patch when applied to the skin.

Product

Electronic Health Record (EHR)

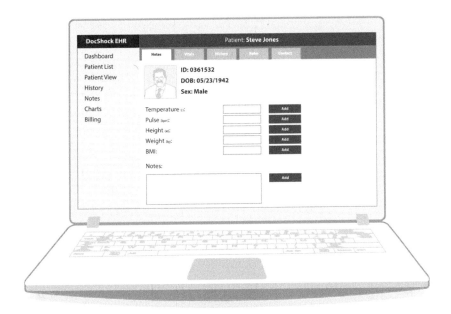

FIGURE 12.22   An electronic health record (EHR).

In many cases, the electronic health record (EHR) is a digital version of the venerable patient chart, expanded to include many other functions related to patient care and billing (Figure 12.22). An EHR might provide health-care professionals with a patient's vital signs over an extended time period, medical procedure records, medication records, and a schedule of appointments (past and future). An EHR usually runs on a healthcare facility's central computer that sends data to, and receives data from, a local digital appliance (e.g., smartphone, mobile tablet, desktop computer). Users include healthcare professionals such as technicians, nurses, therapists, and physicians, as well as those performing supporting roles, including facility managers and the people who handle patient and insurance company billing. Use environments include various points of patient care, such as an emergency department, intensive care unit, and business management offices.

Use Error

ENTERED WEIGHT IN POUNDS INSTEAD OF KILOGRAMS

Two nurses entered the returning patient's weight in pounds (lb) instead of kilograms (kg).

One nurse said that she "blanked" and read the screen's label as pounds instead of kilograms. She said, "I glanced at the screen and was sure the units were in pounds. Now that I look closer, I see it's in kilograms."

The other nurse who erred said that she would never make the same mistake when working in the clinic. She commented, "I think that working with the software in this conference room kind of put me in an at-home frame of mind. At home, like everyone else, I think in pounds. Kind of like when you weigh yourself in the morning on the bathroom scale."

Potential harm

✦ Various harms related to the delivery of weight-based therapies. Medication overdose is one such harm.

Root Cause #1

SMALL TEXT

The EHR displays the units of measure for weight using small text (8 point), which limits its legibility and conspicuity (Figure 12.23).

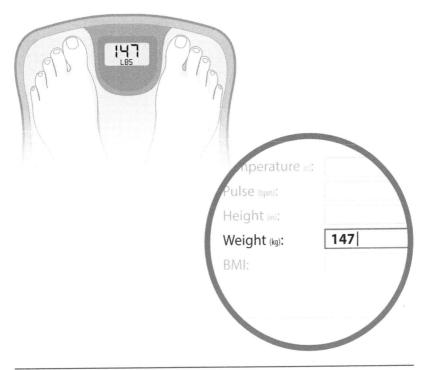

FIGURE 12.23   The weight unit's label (i.e., "kg") is relatively small.

Root Cause #2

RELIANCE ON USER TO DETECT INCORRECT WEIGHT ENTRY

For returning patients, the EHR does not provide feedback when there has been a dramatic (e.g., more than two times) change in weight since the previous data entry. Also, the EHR does not present the data in a form, such as a weight-over-time graph, that would be likely to draw the user's attention to the data entry error. Consequently, the EHR relies on the user to review the patient weight entry and confirm its accuracy.

Suggested Mitigations

ENLARGE UNITS OF MEASURE

Enlarge the units of measure to approximately the same size as the weight value.

ADD AN ALERT

Alert the user, perhaps using a dialog box, when there is an extraordinary weight gain or loss that very likely is due to data entry based on the wrong unit of measure. This suggested mitigation is specific to returning patients (i.e., patients with more than one weight entry).

ADD A GRAPH

Show the latest weight measurement on a graph that also presents previous measurements, thereby exposing a gross data entry error, such as inputting weight in pounds as opposed to kilograms (Figure 12.24).

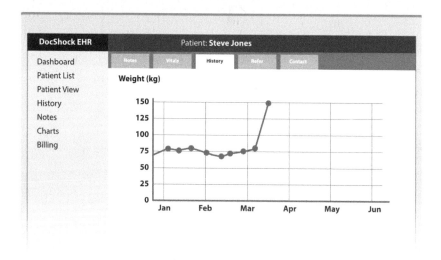

FIGURE 12.24 The revised EHR screen includes a graph that presents the patient's weight over time, as entered in the EHR.

Product

Syringe Infusion Pump

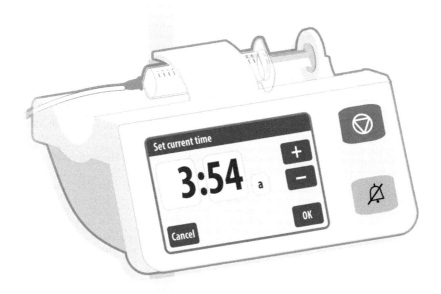

FIGURE 12.25   A syringe infusion pump.

A syringe infusion pump is a small volume infusion pump (Figure 12.25). It infuses fluids (e.g., a pain control medication) over time by pressing the plunger of a syringe at a precise rate over a specified number of hours, thereby expelling fluid into an infusion tube connected to a patient's intravenous access (i.e., a needle or catheter placed through the skin and into a vein). Nurses typically operate syringe infusion pumps in various advanced care settings. Anesthesiologists and nurse anesthetists operate the devices in operating rooms. Even laypersons may be trained to use a syringe pump at home—to deliver pain medication, for example. User tasks include activating the device, programming an infusion, loading a filled syringe into the pump, priming the infusion line, starting and then monitoring the infusion, disconnecting the patient, removing/replacing an empty syringe, and deactivating the device.

Use Error

SET WRONG TIME OF DAY (AM/PM REVERSAL)

The participant set the programmable infusion pump's internal clock to the correct 12-hour time, but did not switch the clock from AM to PM. Specifically, he set the internal clock to 3:54 AM rather than 3:54 PM.

The participant reported the following: "I didn't even notice the 'a' label indicating AM. It's so small that it just doesn't get your attention."

Potential harm

✦ Medication overdose due to medication delivery for too long a duration

✦ Medication underdose due to medication delivery for too short a duration

Root Cause #1

INCONSPICUOUS AM/PM LABEL

The time setting screen indicates AM and PM times using the single letters "a" and "p," respectively. Moreover, the screen displays the "a" or "p" in small (8-point), lowercase text. The small text size and the label's abbreviated lowercase format make the label relatively inconspicuous (Figure 12.26).

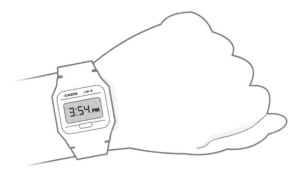

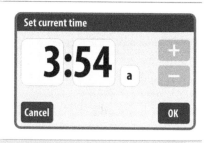

FIGURE 12.26 The "a" label on the "Set current time" screen was not sufficiently conspicuous to capture the participant's attention.

Root Cause #2

LACK OF CONFIRMATION

The infusion pump does not require the user to confirm the internal clock setting. Rather, users must detect an error in the time of day by noticing that the time is set to the incorrect 12-hour time period (e.g., "a" rather than "p") in the time displayed on the main screen.

Root Cause #3

DEFAULT SETTING

The infusion pump defaults to displaying the time of day as an AM setting. The user must highlight the "a" and use the adjustment keys to switch it to "p." As such, users can set a time and then neglect to review and, if necessary, adjust the AM/PM setting.

Suggested Mitigations

MAKE AM/PM LABEL MORE CONSPICUOUS

Display AM and PM in a non-abbreviated, uppercase format and in larger, more visible text (e.g., 18-point, matching the time of day).

ADD SUPPLEMENTAL TEXT

Supplement the time of day (including AM and PM) with one of the following descriptors (Figure 12.27):

Early/mid/late
Morning/afternoon/evening

ADD CONFIRMATION SCREEN

Add a screen requiring the user to confirm that the set time matches the actual time of day. Moreover, remind the user to check that the time is properly set as AM versus PM (Figure 12.28).

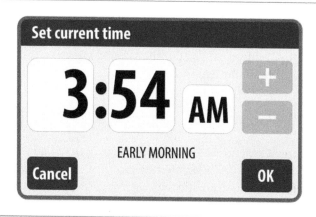

FIGURE 12.27 The revised screen includes a larger, non-abbreviated label and indicates the time of day (i.e., early morning).

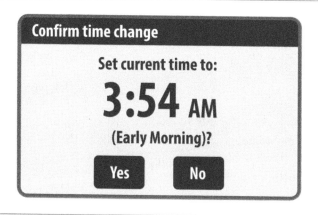

FIGURE 12.28 The additional screen prompts the user to confirm the time change.

Product
Surgical Warming Blanket

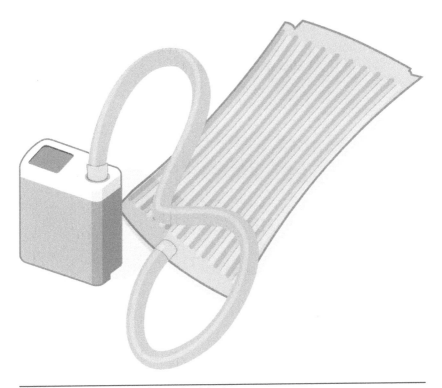

FIGURE 12.29   A surgical warming blanket.

A surgical warming blanket is designed to maintain a surgical patient's normothermic state (i.e., body temperature of 98.6°F) and prevent hypothermia (becoming too cold) (Figure 12.29). During a surgical case, a scrub nurse or other surgical team member will place a warming blanket over the patient's body, making adjustments depending on the patient's temperature control needs and surgical site. The patient is usually anesthetized. Typically, the warming blanket is a single-use, paper-based product that unfolds from a compact unit the size of a book to a billowing form that can cover the patient.

A rolling heater unit, which is usually trash bin sized, delivers thermostatically controlled air to the blanket via a flexible hose. Users might receive in-service training to operate the device, or they might learn on the job.

Use Error

DID NOT ATTACH HOSE TO BLANKET

One nurse did not attach the warming unit's hose to the warming blanket. Rather, she placed the hose tip under the blanket. She later explained that she misunderstood how the product worked. She said, "The first time I used it, I looked at the instructions, but I figured that you should spread the blanket over the patient to hold in the warm air from the heater hose. So, I put the hose under the blanket between the patient's knees so it wouldn't fall to the floor" (Figure 12.30).

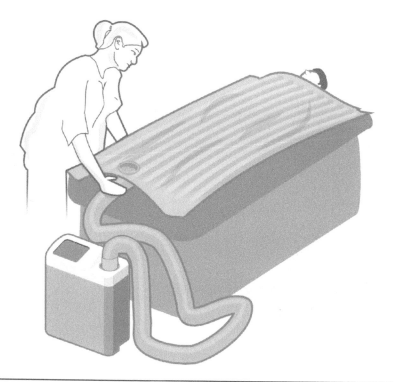

FIGURE 12.30   The participant positioned the hose under the blanket.

Potential harms
+ Skin burn
+ Hypothermia

Root Cause #1
INCONSPICUOUS CONNECTOR

The hose–blanket connector is relatively inconspicuous because it lies flat against the blanket, is not labeled, and has the same medium-blue color as the blanket (Figure 12.31).

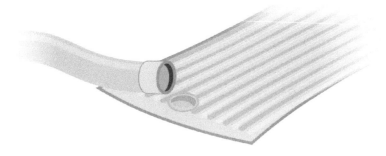

FIGURE 12.31   The hose–blanket connector blends in with the blanket, leading the participant to overlook the connector.

Root Cause #2
UNDERSPECIFIED IFU GRAPHIC

The IFU includes a graphic illustrating how users should connect the warming unit's hose to the blanket, but this graphic does not clearly depict the location of the blanket connector (i.e., inlet). Moreover, the graphic does not show that the hose connects to the blanket, which could lead users to assume they should position the open hose underneath the blanket (Figure 12.32).

Suggested Mitigations
INCREASE CONNECTOR'S CONSPICUITY

Make the hose-to-blanket connector more visually conspicuous, potentially by making both of the components a color that functionally associates them but also distinguishes them from the blue blanket. Also, add a text label near the connection inlet, such as "hose connector." Consider further highlighting the connection inlet by adding an illustration of the warming unit's hose next to the inlet or adding graphical arrowheads that point to the inlet.

REVISE GRAPHIC

Modify the IFU's graphic to show the heater hose connected to the blanket, rather than just placed under it. Include a close-up view of the connection.

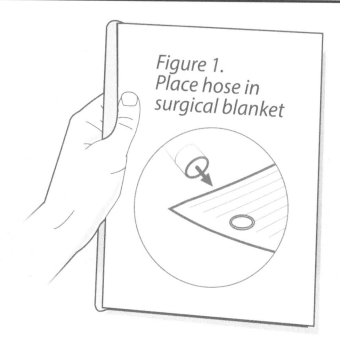

FIGURE 12.32   The graphic does not show the hose connected to the blanket.

Product
Urinary Catheter

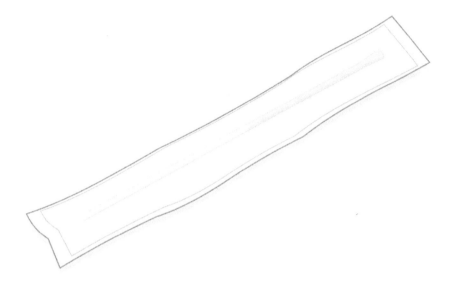

FIGURE 12.33   A urinary catheter.

A urinary catheter is a tube placed into the body to drain urine from the bladder (Figure 12.33). The device may be placed by a healthcare professional (e.g., nurse) or by the patient/layperson, the latter being most common for most types of catheters. Interactions with the device include removing it from its package without causing contamination, inserting it through the urinary meatus and urinary sphincter to reach the bladder, and then reversing the process after draining the bladder. Sometimes users will connect the catheter to a collection bag, as opposed to having it deposit urine directly into a toilet. Laypersons might have a wide range of physical and mental impairments. For example, a user who has paraplegia might have limited hand strength and dexterity. As such, he might choose to perform handling tasks using his teeth (i.e., biting the package to create resistance necessary to pull on a tear strip's tab to open the outer package).

Use Error

FOLDED CATHETERS

Participants were presented with the scenario of preparing to spend the next 8 hours away from home and, as such, needing to bring along a sufficient number of urinary catheters. One participant grasped two catheters and folded them to one-quarter of their normal length so that he could store the catheters in his jacket pocket. Another participant placed four catheters into a backpack, bending them at the approximate one-third points to fit them inside completely.

Both participants reported that they folded the catheters to make them easier to carry. However, bending a catheter creates kinks in its tubing. After the user unfolds the catheter and removes it from its packaging, the tubing often remains kinked, which can impede urine flow (Figure 12.34).

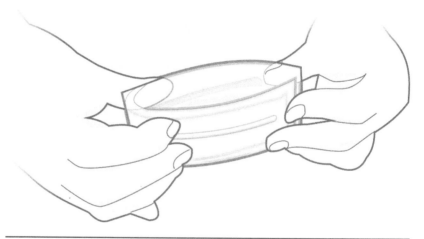

FIGURE 12.34   The participants folded the catheters when storing them.

Potential harms

✦ Incomplete bladder emptying leading to infection
✦ Wasted catheter

Root Cause #1

CATHETER PACKAGING IS NOT SUFFICIENTLY COMPACT

The individual catheters are not packaged in a form that enables users to carry them in usual sizes of storage compartments, such as pockets or backpacks.

Specifically, the catheters are straight, rather than coiled, decreasing users' ability to store them in relatively small areas.

Root Cause #2

RELIANCE ON USER TO KNOW NOT TO FOLD CATHETER

Neither the catheter package nor the package insert instruct (or warn) against folding the catheters. Moreover, the package insert does not explain that folding the catheter can introduce kinks that might persist when extending the catheter at a later point in time.

Suggested Mitigation

REDESIGN PACKAGING

Package the catheter in a coiled form that is not prone to kinking, thereby making the catheter sufficiently compact to store in pockets and other compact containers (Figure 12.35).

FIGURE 12.35   The revised design features a coiled catheter.

Product
Hemodialysis Machine

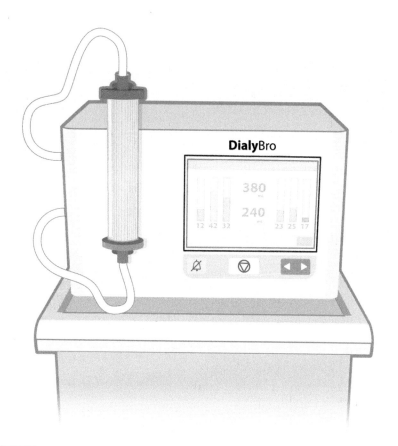

FIGURE 12.36   A hemodialysis machine.

A hemodialysis machine filters a patient's blood to remove excess water and waste products when the kidneys are damaged, dysfunctional, or removed (Figure 12.36). Such machines are traditionally found in hospitals and clinics dedicated to delivering dialysis to patients. However, hemodialysis machines can now be found in the home as well. In professional care settings, the users include dialysis nurses and technicians. In the home, the users include the dialysis patient and caregivers, who might include adult children, adult friends, and partners. Self-treating patients might have a wide range of physical and mental disabilities, but none so severe that it would preclude independent device use. Typical tasks include setting up the machine for use by connecting fluids via multiple tubes, entering or confirming a prescription (e.g., remove 2 liters of fluid over 5 hours), starting and monitoring a treatment, and completing the process by shutting down the machine and performing the necessary cleanup and recycling tasks.

Use Error
DID NOT COUNTER-ROTATE BLOOD TUBE

One participant did not counter-rotate the blood tube before twisting it onto the dialyzer. Consequently, the blood tube kinked at about 5 cm above the point of connection. The participant reportedly did not notice the kink (Figure 12.37).

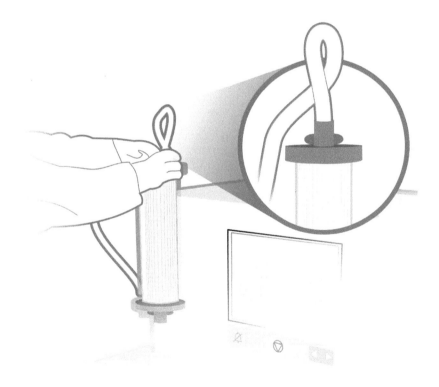

FIGURE 12.37   The blood tube kinked because the participant did not counter-rotate the tube.

Potential harms

✦ Hemolysis*

Root Cause #1

TUBE-DIALYZER CONNECTION RELIES ON USER TO COUNTER-ROTATE

The mechanics of the tube-dialyzer connection rely on the user to counter-rotate the tube before twisting it on to the dialyzer. Specifically, users must counter-rotate a blood tube up to one full turn—an arguably awkward motion—before then twisting the tube on to the dialyzer. Attaching the tube to the dialyzer without counter-rotating it first might torque the tube in a manner that causes it to kink.

Suggested Mitigations

REVISE CONNECTION

Implement a tube-dialyzer connection that does not require the user to counter-rotate the blood tube prior to connecting it to the dialyzer.

ADD A KINKED TUBING ALARM

Implement a means to detect tube kinks prior to the point that a persisting kink could cause hemolysis.

---

* Hemolysis is the destruction of red blood cells, which releases hemoglobin into the plasma and consequently reduces the amount of oxygen in the blood.

Product
Ultrasonic Nebulizer

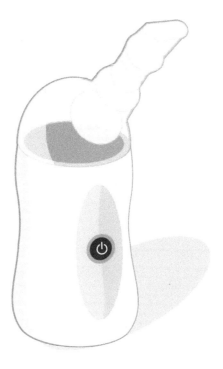

FIGURE 12.38   An ultrasonic nebulizer.

An ultrasonic nebulizer uses high-frequency vibrations to turn liquid medication into a very fine mist (i.e., an aerosol) that can be inhaled into the lungs
to treat respiratory diseases such as asthma, chronic obstructive pulmonary
disease (COPD), and cystic fibrosis (Figure 12.38). The device is typically
used in the home by laypersons and in clinical settings (e.g., emergency
department) by respiratory therapists and nurses. User tasks may include
assembling the device, adding medication into a reservoir, starting the
device, inserting the mouthpiece into the patient's mouth, the patient inhaling the medicinal aerosol for a specified period of time, ending treatment,
disassembling the device, cleaning the components, and storing them properly. Laypersons might have physical impairments, such as arthritis, that
complicate manual manipulation of device components.

Use Error

DID NOT DISINFECT COMPONENTS

Presented with the use scenario that the nebulizer had been used "two days in a row without special maintenance," two participants proceeded to perform the usual daily rinse, rather than performing the required disinfection. Specifically, they held the disassembled components under warm water for a few seconds rather than disinfecting the components by either soaking them in a vinegar and water solution for 60 minutes or placing them in boiling water for 10 minutes.

Potential harms
- ✦ Bacterial infection
- ✦ Medication underdose

Root Cause #1

RELIANCE ON USER TO REALIZE REQUIREMENT TO DISINFECT COMPONENTS

The nebulizer has no label or other form of reminder to help users recognize that the device requires disinfection on every other day of use. Instead, users must recollect the intermittent need for nebulizer disinfection after learning of this requirement from the nebulizer's IFU.

Root Cause #2

INCONSPICUOUS INSTRUCTION

The IFU content that directs users to disinfect the nebulizer's components is relatively inconspicuous, separated from the IFU's primary, step-by-step guidance. The disinfection requirement is also presented within a densely packed paragraph of seemingly supplemental information. Moreover, the text is small (8 point), has no highlighting that might draw the user's attention, and lacks the graphical reinforcement that typifies the primary, step-by-step guidance (Figure 12.39).

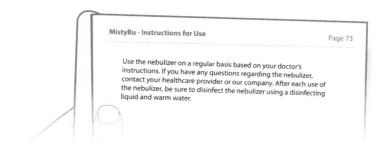

FIGURE 12.39   The IFU presents the instruction to disinfect the nebulizer in a section containing supplemental information.

Suggested Mitigations

ADD LABEL

Add a label to the device that reminds users to disinfect the device in accordance with a prescribed frequency, in this case every other treatment day (Figure 12.40).

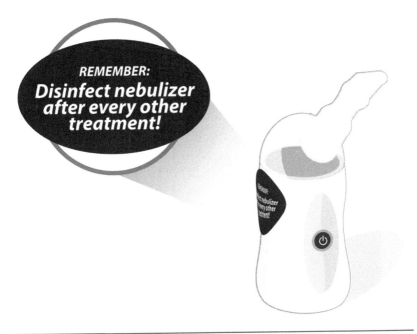

FIGURE 12.40   The new label is a conspicuous reminder to disinfect the nebulizer every two days.

MODIFY IFU

Make the IFU text pertaining to intermittent disinfection more conspicuous and reinforce this text with a graphical depiction of component disinfection. Furthermore, embed the disinfection information in the procedural instructions, rather than presenting it as supplemental information (Figure 12.41).

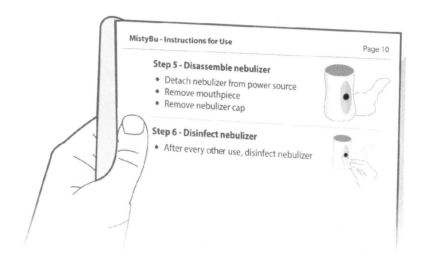

FIGURE 12.41   The revised instructions include a separate step for disinfecting the nebulizer.

Product

Ventricular Assist Device (VAD)

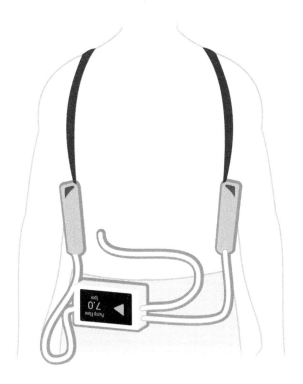

FIGURE 12.42   A ventricular assist device (VAD).

A ventricular assist device is a system of components that serve to boost blood flow in people who have weakened hearts (Figure 12.42). In most cases, the system includes an implantable pump, external power sources (e.g., multiple batteries), a pump controller/computer, and various cables and other accessories. The device normally serves as a "bridge to transplant," meaning that it provides circulatory support to a patient until a donor heart becomes available. Users include the clinicians and other members of a VAD team who perform the implantation procedure (including programming) and the patient and supporting caregivers. VAD team members are highly trained at VAD procedures, which can span many hours at a time. Patient/caregiver tasks include changing batteries and responding to alarm conditions. Such patients may have different degrees of debilitation, but generally get healthier once placed on the therapy.

Use Error
DID NOT FULLY CONNECT BATTERY PACK

Two nurses failed to connect the battery pack to the VAD securely. Although both nurses inserted the battery pack into its slot in the VAD, they did not press the pack firmly and far enough into the slot to make a secure connection that would enable the proper transfer of power. Consequently, the VAD lost power.

One nurse explained, "I thought the battery was all the way in place because it looked right. It was flush with the device." The other nurse stated, "There was nothing telling me that I hadn't pushed it in far enough, so I assumed I did it correctly."

Potential harms

+ Loss of mechanical circulatory support, leading to insufficient blood flow
+ Thromboembolism (i.e., blood clot) if device is restarted after being inactive for several minutes

Root Cause #1
BATTERY APPEARS FLUSH WITH DEVICE WHEN INSERTED INCOMPLETELY

In its proper, connected position, the battery is recessed approximately 5 mm into the device housing. However, both participants assumed that the battery was fully inserted when the battery was flush with the device housing because the battery had a "finished" appearance; they noted that a certain amount of protrusion from or indentation into the housing would have looked "unfinished." Consequently, these participants did not press the battery deep enough into the housing to create a secure connection (Figure 12.43).

Root Cause #2
LACK OF LOCAL FEEDBACK

The VAD does not provide salient feedback when the user inserts the battery properly. Rather, it provides only onscreen feedback that is likely not within the user's line of sight while he or she inserts the battery into its slot.

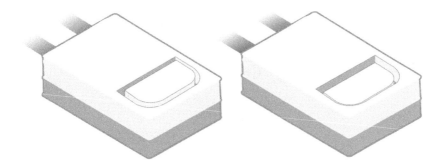

FIGURE 12.43 The battery is flush with the housing when it is inserted incorrectly (left) and recessed when it is fully inserted (right).

Suggested Mitigations

REDESIGN BATTERY COMPARTMENT

Redesign the battery compartment so that the battery looks definitively out of place unless the user fully inserts it. For example, the slot could be engineered to cause the battery to stick out at least 1 cm if it is not inserted properly.

ADD "BATTERY CONNECTED" INDICATOR

Add a bi-colored LED directly above the battery slot that is green when the battery is properly energized (i.e., the battery is connected) and red when it is not.

Product

Auto-Injector

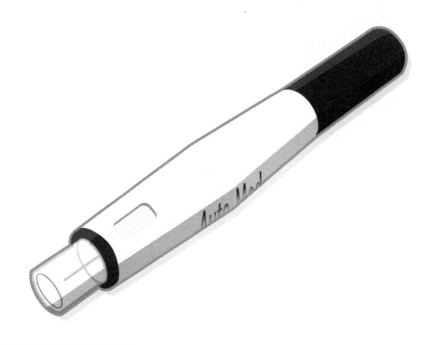

FIGURE 12.44 An auto-injector.

An auto-injector is a drug delivery device designed to deliver a single dose of a particular drug (Figure 12.44). As such, users do not have to set a dose. Rather, they just press the auto-injector against a body part to automatically actuate it, or they actuate the injection manually by pressing a button. Most users are laypersons, although some auto-injectors are used by healthcare professionals. Laypersons might have various medical conditions associated with the injection therapy, such as rheumatoid arthritis, multiple sclerosis (MS), diabetes, Parkinson's disease, hemophilia, and growth hormone deficiency that pose an array of physical and mental limitations on device handling.

Use Error

DID NOT INSPECT DRUG

Two participants did not inspect the fluid reservoir to confirm that the drug was free of defects and suitable for use. Consequently, the participant did not notice that the drug was discolored (yellowed) and contained particulates. One participant commented, "I wasn't exactly sure where to look. I figured it was probably OK to use." The other participant commented, "I completely forgot to check it. I remember reading something about checking the drug to see if it was OK, but then it slipped my mind. It didn't seem particularly important."

Potential harms

- ✦ Systemic infection
- ✦ Local infection at injection site

Root Cause #1

SMALL INSPECTION WINDOW

The two inspection windows, located on opposite sides of the auto-injector's barrel, are relatively small (5 mm × 2.5 mm rectangle), making them rather inconspicuous and unlikely to induce users to check the fluid for defects. The inspection windows become even less conspicuous when the user rotates the barrel such that the windows face away from the user (Figure 12.45).

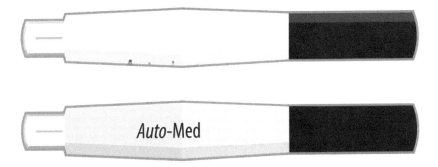

FIGURE 12.45 The auto-injector's inspection window is relatively small (top) and the window is not visible from all angles (bottom).

Root Cause #2
NO EXPLANATION OF CONSEQUENCE

The IFU directs the user to check the drug for discoloration and particulates. However, the document does not state the consequence of injecting a contaminated drug. Consequently, the instruction to check the drug clarity is less likely to compel users to perform the inspection or, in some cases, even remember to perform it.

Suggested Mitigations
INCREASE INSPECTION WINDOW CONSPICUITY

Design the inspection window to be more conspicuous by one or more of the following means: increase the window size, add a colored outline around the windows, and add a label instructing users to inspect the drug (Figure 12.46).

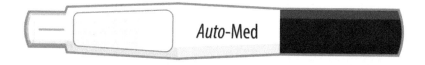

FIGURE 12.46 The revised auto-injector features a larger window that is outlined in blue.

STATE CONSEQUENCE OF INJECTING CONTAMINATED DRUG

Continue directing users to inspect the fluid for discoloration and particulates. In addition, state the consequences of injecting a contaminated drug to help increase compliance with the instruction (Figure 12.47).

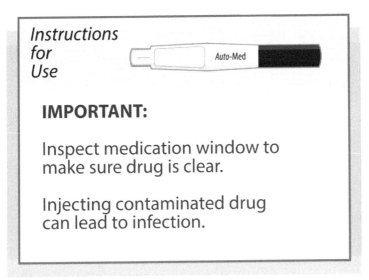

Instructions for Use

IMPORTANT:

Inspect medication window to make sure drug is clear.

Injecting contaminated drug can lead to infection.

FIGURE 12.47   The revised instruction indicates that injecting a contaminated drug can lead to infection.

Product

Stretcher

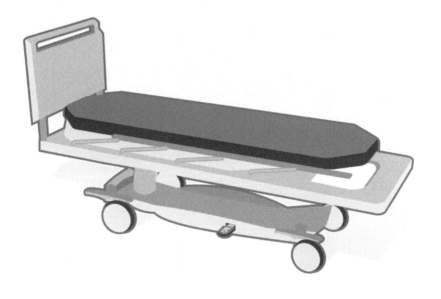

FIGURE 12.48   A stretcher.

A stretcher is a type of hospital bed that is frequently used to transport patients within medical care facilities, as well as the primary bed in several care environments such as emergency departments (Figure 12.48). As compared to hospital beds that reside in patient rooms, stretchers are used on a short-term basis (e.g., up to a few hours). Users include transport personnel (e.g., "candy stripers," orderlies, nurse assistants) and various other clinical staff (e.g., physicians, nurses) who may need to gain access to the patient by lowering the stretcher's side rails or adjusting the stretcher to enable CPR delivery.

Use Error

DID NOT PLACE STRETCHER IN CPR MODE

One nurse did not pull the dedicated blue metal CPR lever before commencing CPR on the simulated patient. Therefore, the stretcher was not in the prescribed flat position and fully inflated state. Rather, the stretcher was configured such that the simulated patient's head and knees were raised. Moreover, the air mattress remained somewhat soft, rather than inflated to maximum pressure to provide a firmer foundation for CPR delivery.

Instead of pulling the CPR lever, the participant manually lowered the stretcher's head and knee sections to a horizontal position using the primary position controls, and then started CPR with the air mattress still on a "soft" setting. Consequently, the nurse's chest compressions caused the simulated patient to sink into the air mattress repeatedly in a manner that would likely reduce the compressions' effectiveness.

The nurse, who as planned did not receive training on the stretcher's use before participating in the test session, commented, "I was not aware the stretcher had a special control to configure it for CPR. That's a nice feature, but you'd need training to know that the lever is down there. Maybe it could be up higher between the head rail and the side rail."

Potential harms
+ Delayed cardiopulmonary resuscitation
+ Ineffective cardiopulmonary resuscitation

Root Cause #1
INCONSPICUOUS CPR LEVER

The CPR lever is located at a relatively low position on the stretcher's frame, disassociated from the stretcher's primary controls. As such, the nurse did not notice the CPR lever. Therefore, she was unaware that the bed had a CPR mode that could be activated by pulling on the CPR lever (Figure 12.49).

Suggested Mitigations
PLACE CPR LEVER IN CONSPICUOUS LOCATION

Place the CPR lever in a location where it is likely to be noticed and is easier to reach, such as higher on the stretcher's frame. Ensure the lever is in a location that is unlikely to be covered by sheets or blankets.

COLOR CPR LEVER

Color the CPR lever red to make it conspicuous and to identify it as an emergency control (Figure 12.50).

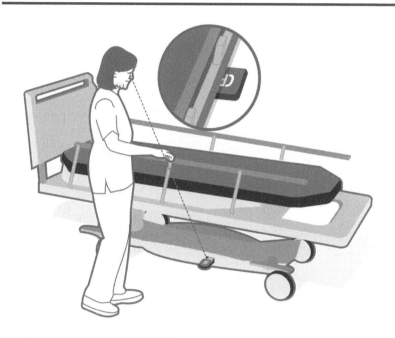

FIGURE 12.49 The user does not have a clear view of the CPR lever due to the lever's position on the frame.

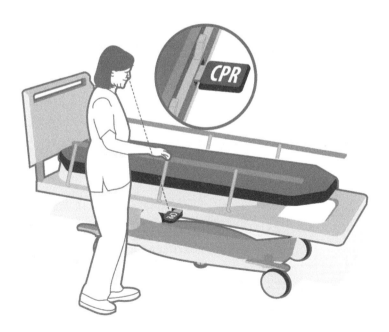

FIGURE 12.50 A red lever that is positioned higher on the stretcher's frame is more likely to capture the user's attention.

Product

Smartphone Application: Insulin Bolus Calculator

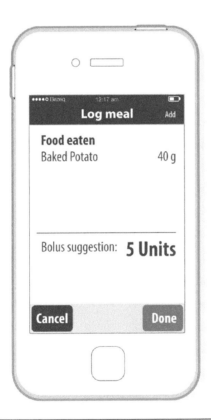

FIGURE 12.51   A smartphone application with an insulin bolus calculator.

An insulin bolus calculator is a smartphone-based tool that enables people with diabetes to calculate the amount of insulin they should administer to cover a meal they are preparing to eat (Figure 12.51). The calculator might be used in conjunction with an insulin delivery device, such as a wearable pump or a pen-injector. User inputs might include the types of food eaten during a recent meal or perhaps just the number of carbohydrates consumed, the user's current and target blood glucose levels, insulin sensitivity level, the amount of "insulin on board," and more. A young individual who has excellent glycemic control might not have any particular impairments, while others might have some degree of physical and mental impairment associated with diabetes, co-morbidities, and being outside their target blood glucose range (i.e., experiencing hypoglycemia or hyperglycemia).

Use Error

DID NOT ENTER ALL CARBOHYDRATES

Participants used the application to determine an appropriate meal time insulin bolus based on a list of meal contents. One participant used the application's food library to determine the number of grams of carbohydrate that he would have consumed in the example meal. He determined the correct number of grams for a large baked potato (40 grams), but did not look up the carbohydrates in the medium-sized dinner roll (15 grams). Consequently, he determined that he had consumed 40 rather than 55 grams of carbohydrate. He entered 40 grams into the bolus calculator to obtain a bolus recommendation of five units of insulin, which was less than the necessary seven units.

The test participant commented, "I intended to include the bread but once I found the carbs for the potato, I forgot to keep going and just hit the "Done" button. Maybe it made a difference that I didn't really eat the meal but was just simulating it for you guys."

Potential harm
 + Hyperglycemia

Root Cause #1

BUTTON PLACEMENT

The "Add" button's placement in the screen's top-right corner can be overlooked; this position on a screen is generally considered less conspicuous than other positions (e.g., top left, bottom right). The user's attention is likely to progress from the top of the screen toward the carbohydrate entry field in the screen's middle, and then progress to the "Done" button at the screen's bottom. As such, the "Done" button is a "call to action" that could lead users to forget to use the "Add" button to look up and enter additional carbohydrate values (Figure 12.52).

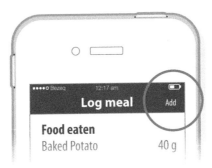

FIGURE 12.52   The "Add" button is relatively inconspicuous.

Root Cause #2
TEST ARTIFACT

The participant had not actually consumed a meal that included both a baked potato and a dinner roll. This might have contributed to his overlooking the need to account for the dinner roll in the bolus calculation exercise.

Suggested Mitigations
RELOCATE "ADD" BUTTON

Place the "Add" button where the user is likely to view it in the natural progression of visual attention from the top of the screen to the bottom.

RENAME "ADD" BUTTON

Rename the "Add" button to "Add more carbs" to present a more explicit call to action (Figure 12.53).

ADD CARBOHYDRATE SUMMARY SCREEN

Add a screen that lists all of the carbohydrate entries and requires the user to confirm that the list is complete and accurate before the user can view a recommended insulin bolus value.

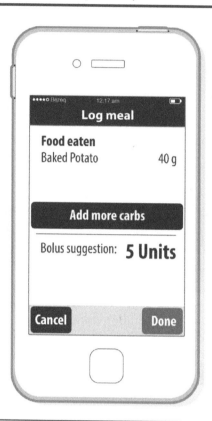

FIGURE 12.53 The redesigned screen includes a more descriptive button title. Additionally, the "Add more carbs" button is positioned in the screen's center.

Product

Naloxone Nasal Spray

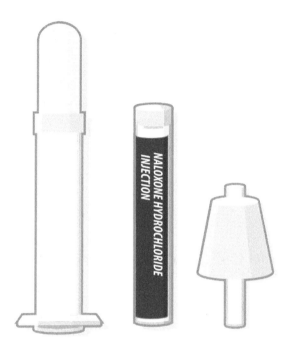

FIGURE 12.54   A Naloxone nasal spray.

Naloxone is a drug used to treat patients experiencing an opioid (e.g., Oxycodone, heroin) overdose (Figure 12.54). Users may administer Naloxone as a nasal spray, splitting a dose between two nostrils for more complete medication absorption. To date, most users have been first responders (e.g., paramedics, emergency medical technicians) who encounter someone who is likely to be unconscious and perhaps close to death. First responders are trained to use the device. User tasks include assembling the device from a set of components, dispensing half portions of the total dose into each of the patient's nostrils, and then disposing of the device properly.

Use Error

DID NOT SPRAY NALOXONE INTO BOTH NOSTRILS

Three participants sprayed the entire dose of Naloxone into a single nostril, rather than splitting the dose evenly between the simulated patient's nostrils. Specifically, these participants inserted the cone into one nostril and then pressed steadily on the syringe's plunger until all of the medication was delivered.

Immediately after committing this same use error, two out of the three participants spontaneously commented that they forgot to split the dose between the two nostrils, but that it was too late to do anything about it. The other participant commented, "I know you are supposed to split the dose between nostrils, but I figured it was fine to deliver the entire dose at once. You administer it faster that way."

Potential harms

✦ Underdose, leading to patient death due to opioid overdose[*]

Root Cause #1

RELIANCE ON USER TO SPLIT DOSE

The nasal spray's label does not direct the user to split the dose between two nostrils. Consequently, the product relies on the user to intuit that he or she must administer half of the medication into one nostril and half into the other.

Root Cause #2

INSTRUCTIONS DO NOT EXPLAIN BENEFIT OF DOSE SPLITTING

Although the IFU directs the user to split the dose between two nostrils, it does not explain why doing so is clinically beneficial. As such, some users might not consider dose splitting to be an important step and decide to skip it.

---

[*] When the user administers Naloxone to only one nostril, the nasal surface area for medication absorption is less than if the user administers medication to both nostrils. Consequently, medication delivery via one nostril can be fatal because the patient does not absorb enough Naloxone to treat the opioid overdose.

Root Cause #3
NO CLEAR HALF-WAY POINT

The Naloxone nasal spray enables the user to deliver the entire dose in a single action (i.e., pressing steadily on the syringe plunger until the entire dose has been delivered to the patient). For example, the nasal spray does not provide feedback that half the dose has been delivered, so the user should switch nostrils.

Suggested Mitigations
REVISE LABELING

Add an on-product label directing the user to administer half of the dose into each nostril. Additionally, add more detail to the syringe gradations to indicate the half-way point (Figure 12.55).

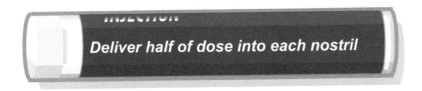

FIGURE 12.55 The additional on-product label prompts the user to split the dose between both nostrils.

Add a warning to the IFU that advises against delivering the entire dose into one nostril. Also, explain the benefit of delivering a half-dose into each nostril to improve compliance among users who might not otherwise follow the instruction.

ADD TACTILE FEEDBACK

Develop a syringe that provides tactile feedback when the user reaches the half-way point, thereby signaling the need to switch to the second nostril.

Product

Enteral Feeding Pump

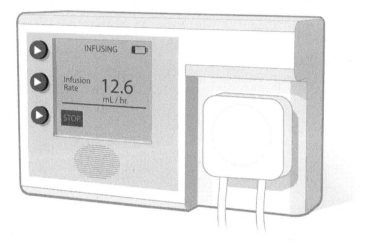

FIGURE 12.56 An enteral feeding pump.

An enteral feeding pump delivers enteral nutrition to people who cannot obtain adequate nutrition or hydration orally (Figure 12.56). Nutritional fluids pass from the pump through a tube and into the patient. The tube may be percutaneous (passing through the skin) or be passed through the nasal passages to the stomach. Feedings may be delivered by healthcare professionals, such as nurses and assistants working in a long-term care facility, or by patients and their caregivers who use the pump at home. User tasks include installing a disposable tubing set into the pump, programming the pump to deliver a specified amount of enteral nutrition, connecting the pump's outflow tube to the patient's feeding tube, and starting and then monitoring the feeding process. Users may occasionally need to respond to device alarms. Some healthcare professionals might have extensive training to use the device but others might not. Patients are likely to be trained to operate the pump's basic features, but might face challenges posed by physical and/ or mental impairments.

Use Error
DID NOT HEAR ALARM

Two participants did not detect the low battery alarm, which the enteral feeding pump emitted steadily as a square waveform at a frequency of 4000 Hz and at a volume of 80 dB (i.e., a high-pitched, periodic beep).

Notably, both participants reported being somewhat "hard of hearing," especially with respect to high-pitched sounds.

Potential harms
+ Delay of therapy
+ Incomplete feeding

Root Cause #1
SOUND FREQUENCY TOO HIGH

The alarm was not audible to the participants because its frequency was too high. Both individuals had high-frequency hearing loss, an age-related condition called presbycusis*. Accordingly, these participants did not hear the otherwise penetrating alarm tone.

Root Cause #2
SINGLE MODALITY ALARM

The device presents the low battery alarm using a single modality—an auditory alarm—rather than using redundant modalities, such as auditory and visual alarms. As such, the device relies on the user's ability to hear the auditory alarm, which can pose challenges to users with hearing impairments.

Suggested Mitigations
REDUCE ALARM TONE FREQUENCY

Lower the alarm tone frequency from 4000 to 1000 Hz, for example. Moreover, meeting associated alarm standards (e.g., IEC 60601-1-8:2006) might compel a switch to a sound generator that can emit more complex sounds.

---

* As described in ANSI/AAMI HE75:2009/(R)2013, presbycusis is typified by the decreased ability to hear sounds above 2000 Hz, which is common among males in their early 50s and older.

ADD VISUAL ALARM

Add a visual alarm to the device, such as a flashing LED, to increase the likelihood that the low battery alarm captures the user's attention (Figure 12.57).

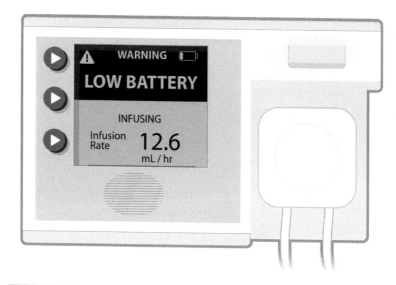

FIGURE 12.57 The redesigned pump features a flashing yellow LED.

Product

Metered Dose Inhaler

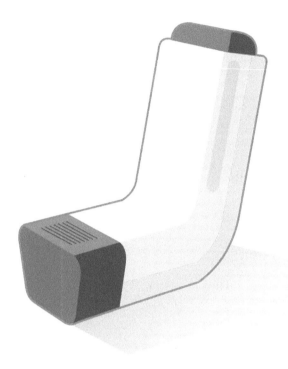

FIGURE 12.58   A metered dose inhaler.

A metered dose inhaler is used to deliver aerosolized medication into the body via the lungs (Figure 12.58). The product is commonly used by people with asthma, including children, adults, and the elderly. User tasks include placing a canister in a meter dose inhaler (when starting therapy or replacing an empty canister), sometimes attaching a spacer, dispensing a dose by pressing on the canister, and exhaling and inhaling at the proper times to receive a full dose. Some users might have impairments influencing their ability to hold the device securely and time their breathing properly.

Use Error

HELD INHALER UPSIDE DOWN

Two participants held the inhaler upside down (i.e., inverted) while attempting to administer a dose of aerosolized medication. Consequently, the participants did not receive the full dose because the inhaler's dose delivery mechanism does not aerosolize the entire drug when the user holds the inhaler upside down.

One test participant stated, "I didn't even notice the 'THIS SIDE UP' label. They should have made it black so it would get your attention." Another participant stated, "The inhaler looks like you should be able to hold it any way you want to. If you have to hold it with this side up, then it should have an arrow on it pointing up or something" (Figure 12.59).

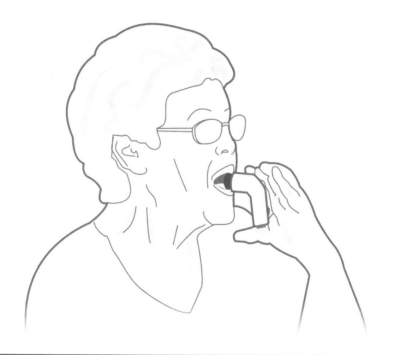

FIGURE 12.59 The participants administered the medication while holding the inhaler upside down.

Potential harms
+ Underdose
+ No dose

Root Cause #1

INSUFFICIENT ORIENTATION CUES

The tube-like inhaler's top and bottom have a nearly identical appearance. Their similarity led the participants to conclude that it did not matter which side faced up when they delivered a dose.

Root Cause #2
INCONSPICUOUS LABEL

The "THIS SIDE UP" text label is molded into the device, resulting in text that does not contrast appreciably against its background. Consequently, the label was relatively inconspicuous and failed to draw the participants' attention.

Suggested Mitigations
PRINT INSTRUCTION ON DEVICE

Print "THIS SIDE UP" in durable, high-contrast text near the inhaler's top (Figure 12.60).

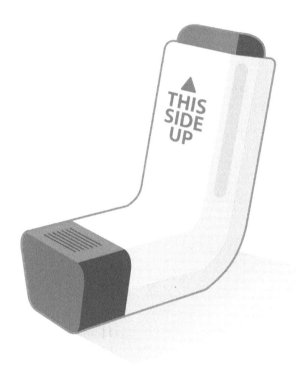

FIGURE 12.60   The redesigned inhaler includes a label indicating the proper orientation.

MODIFY CASE

Consider case modifications (e.g., shape, material, texture, color) that will enable users to more readily differentiate the inhaler's top from its bottom.

Product

Drug Patch Pump

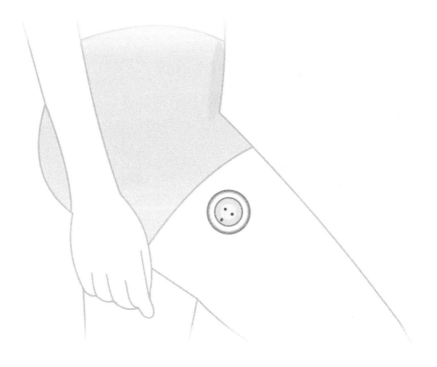

FIGURE 12.61 A drug patch pump.

A patch pump delivers a drug subcutaneously via a cannula inserted into the body (often the abdomen or thigh) (Figure 12.61). Insulin delivery is a common application. Users are primarily laypersons who require drug therapy at a steady rate and/or require a bolus on an as-needed basis. Pharmacists and nurses have more limited interactions with the devices during prescription fulfillment and patient training, respectively. The layperson is expected to prepare an injection site, adhere the device to his or her body, take the necessary steps to trigger cannula insertion, inspect the patch for any problems (e.g., leaking drug, signs of infection), deliver a drug bolus as necessary, and remove and replace the patch at the prescribed interval (e.g., every 3 days). Laypersons might have various medical conditions or co-morbidities associated with the therapy that could pose an array of physical and mental limitations on device handling.

Use Error
INJECTED DRUG INTO WRONG DEVICE PORT

Three participants erroneously injected the drug into the cannula port, rather than into the drug filling port.

One participant reported, "I had to guess which hole I should stick the syringe into. I chose the one that seemed to be closer to the center because I assumed the drug is stored in the middle of the patch."

Another commented, "It would be better if the place for the needle has a label so you would know exactly where to fill the patch pump. Maybe it could have a drawing of a syringe pointing to it. Or, maybe it could have a big colored circle around it and the words 'Fill Here' or something like that."

The other participant reported that he was initially unsure where to inject the drug, so he reviewed the IFU. The participant further explained, "I checked the instructions for help, but the picture of the drug filling port and the cannula port do not look like the actual patch pump, so I still couldn't figure it out."

Potential harms
+ Underdose
+ Delay of therapy
+ Wasted device

Root Cause #1
SIMILAR COMPONENT APPEARANCE

The drug filling port and the cannula port look nearly identical, making them difficult to differentiate. The two ports are approximately 4 mm diameter holes on the patch pump's underside, with location as their only distinguishable difference.

Root Cause #2
LACK OF LABELS

The patch pump does not label the drug filling port or the cannula port. Consequently, the device relies on the user to distinguish between these two components to inject the drug into the correct location (Figure 12.62).

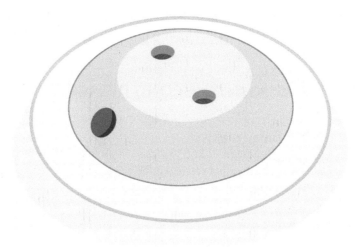

FIGURE 12.62 The drug filling port and the cannula port are not labeled.

Root Cause #3
INACCURATE GRAPHIC

The IFU graphic's depiction of the drug filling port and the cannula port is not representative of the actual device. Specifically, the graphic depicts the two components evenly spaced on the patch. However, the cannula port is near the patch's center and the drug filling port is off center.

Suggested Mitigations
LABEL DRUG FILLING PORT

Clearly identify the drug filling port to increase the likelihood that the user intuits the port's purpose. Options include highlighting it with a bold outline and/or labeling it with an icon and/or text (Figure 12.63).

MAKE CANNULA PORT INACCESSIBLE TO A NEEDLE

Explore opportunities to make the cannula port inaccessible to a needle. In other words, revise it so that a needle cannot be inserted into it.

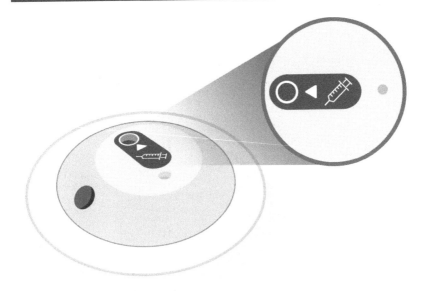

FIGURE 12.63   Labeling the drug filling port with a syringe icon increases the likelihood the user will intuit the port's purpose.

Product

Patient Monitor

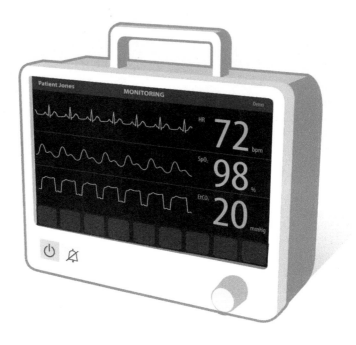

FIGURE 12.64   A patient monitor.

Healthcare professionals use patient monitors to view patient health information in a variety of use environments, such as intensive care units, operating rooms, and emergency rooms (Figure 12.64). Patient monitors are usually placed on a shelf or wall-mounted boom above and to the side of the patient's head. They display vital signs as waveforms and numerical values, and they emit alarms when vital signs go outside healthy ranges. Users include nurses, therapists, and physicians who are unlikely to have significant, uncorrected impairments. They might or might not have received formal training on how to use a particular monitor, but most likely will have used many different types of monitors that have unique user interfaces.

Use Error

USED DEMO OPERATION MODE TO MONITOR PATIENT

Two participants monitored the simulated patient with the patient monitor in demo (i.e., training) mode. The task called for the monitor to begin in demo mode, as though it had been used most recently in a training exercise for new staff. However, the participants did not switch the monitor from demo mode to operation mode before performing the monitoring task. Consequently, the participants mistook the demo data for their patient's vital signs.

During the post-test interview, one participant commented, "I had no idea the monitor was stuck in demo mode. I think it should always start in normal mode or make you confirm whether it should stay in demo mode or not." The participant added, "I probably would have noticed that it was not working correctly if I had hooked it up to a real patient. The vital signs were very stable."

The second participant commented, "I assumed the monitor was in normal mode because that is the mode it was in during the previous task. I'm sure I would have checked the operating mode in a real situation because I always perform a thorough equipment check before my morning cases."

Potential harm(s):
+ Delayed detection and response to various emergency medical conditions

Root Cause #1

INCONSPICUOUS MODE INDICATION

The mode indication is relatively inconspicuous due to its relatively small, 12-point text size and the absence of any other visual characteristics, such as color coding or flashing, which might draw users' attention to the mode indication (Figure 12.65).

Root Cause #2

DEFAULT TO DEMO MODE

Users expected the patient monitor to start up in its normal (i.e., default) operating mode, as opposed to the less frequently used demo mode.

Root Cause #3

TEST ARTIFACT

The use errors might have been induced in part by the artificial test scenario, which called for the test participant to imagine that it had been several days

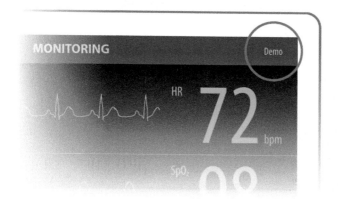

FIGURE 12.65 The "Demo" mode indication is relatively inconspicuous.

since he or she had last performed a case or interacted with the given patient monitor. The previous task could have instilled a mind set that the device was in its normal operating mode because the participants had not switched it into demo mode themselves.

Suggested Mitigations

DEFAULT TO NORMAL OPERATING MODE WITH THE USER'S CONFIRMATION

Make the patient monitor automatically switch back to normal operating mode when the user signals the start of a new patient case. Also, make the monitor start up in its normal operating mode. There is no need for the user to acknowledge the mode change because switching to the normal operating mode does not pose a risk.

INCREASE CONSPICUITY OF DEMO MODE INDICATION

Redesign the demo mode indication to make it more conspicuous and distinguish it from normal operating mode. For example, increase the mode title's text size, contrast its color to the rest of the user interface, and flash the title subtly to draw attention to it, thereby increasing the likelihood that the user recognizes that the device is in demo mode. Additionally, place the "Demo mode" heading on a colored header background to help the users detect the device mode at a glance (Figure 12.66).

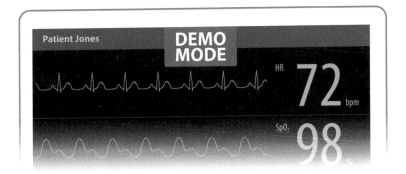

FIGURE 12.66   The updated monitor user interface features a large, red "Demo mode" indicator.

Product

Jet Nebulizer

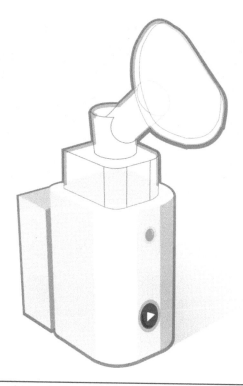

FIGURE 12.67 A jet nebulizer.

A jet nebulizer aerosolizes liquid medication using compressed air or oxygen (Figure 12.67). The patient inhales the mist generated by the nebulizer. Jet nebulizers are often used in urgent care scenarios, such as when a person in respiratory distress seeks more aggressive treatment at a hospital, but the devices are also used in the home. Jet nebulizers usually require some assembly and then dismantling and cleaning after use. The home user might be a layperson with a respiratory ailment or a caregiver (e.g., a parent delivering a treatment to a child). These users might have a range of impairments common in the general population. More importantly, someone who self-administers a treatment might be suffering the effects of reduced oxygen saturation, depending on the cause for the treatment, and feel stressed.

Use Error
DID NOT ADMINISTER FULL DOSE

Believing he had completed the dose, one participant stopped inhaling the medication and removed the nebulizer from his mouth before the nebulizer had delivered the full dose of medication.

Importantly, the participant had not assembled the nebulizer correctly. Specifically, he had attached the mouthpiece upside down. Consequently, the participant could not see the dose progress LEDs because the LEDs were on the side opposite the nebulizer, facing away from him.

During the post-task interview, the participant stated, "I assumed I attached that [mouth] piece correctly because it fit right into the nebulizer. I didn't realize the nebulizer had a progress bar because I couldn't see the lights."

Potential harms
　✦　Underdose

Root Cause #1
MOUTHPIECE CAN BE ATTACHED TWO WAYS

The mouthpiece is keyed to ensure that it points in a line that is orthogonal to the display. However, this makes it possible for the user to orient the mouthpiece 180° opposite the intended direction (Figure 12.68).

Root Cause #2
SINGLE-MODALITY DOSE PROGRESS INDICATOR

The nebulizer indicates the dose's progress using a single modality (six LEDs), rather than using redundant modalities (i.e., both visual and audible indicators). As such, the nebulizer relies on the user's ability to see the LEDs during dose administration, which is not possible if the user assembles the nebulizer such that the LEDs face away from him or her.

Suggested Mitigations
KEYING

Key the mouthpiece so that the user can only insert it in its correct orientation (Figure 12.69).

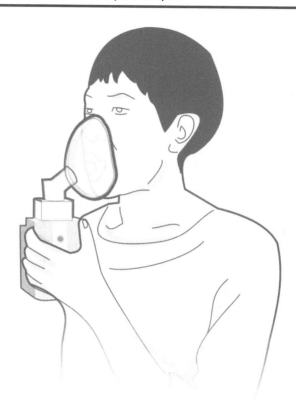

FIGURE 12.68 The mouthpiece can be attached such that the display faces away from the user when he or she administers a dose.

ADD AUDIBLE DOSE PROGRESS INDICATOR

Add an audible indication of dose progress. For example, the nebulizer could emit a single beep as each dose progress LED illuminates and a different "dose complete" beep when the nebulizer has delivered the full dose.

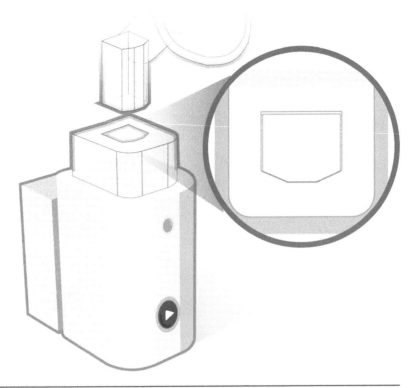

FIGURE 12.69   The revised hardware features a keyed mouthpiece which fits into the nebulizer only in the correct orientation.

Product

Syringe

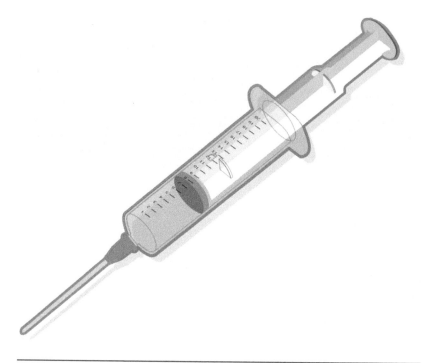

FIGURE 12.70   A syringe.

A syringe consists of a plunger that slides within a hollow barrel (i.e., tube) (Figure 12.70). Many syringes have an attached needle but some have a plastic tip that twists onto tubes with compatible connectors (e.g., Luer-type connectors). Syringes may be prefilled with medication or require the user (e.g., nurse and pharmacist) to draw medication into the syringe from a vial. Sometimes syringes are used to reconstitute lyophilized drug (i.e., powder) into a fluid medication. Interacting with syringes is a basic clinician skill.

Use Error

DREW UP INCORRECT AMOUNT OF DILUENT

The participant drew up 16 mL instead of 14 mL of diluent (0.9% sterile saline used to reconstitute a powered drug). As a result, she reconstituted the drug using more diluent than necessary and ultimately produced the incorrect drug concentration (i.e., the concentration was too weak). The participant commented, "I could barely make out the gray marks on the syringe. It would be better if they were darker. Maybe they should be black or at least a dark gray instead of light gray. They get lost against the reflections in the glass tube."

Potential harms
+ Underdose due to low drug concentration

Root Cause #1

POOR CONTRAST BETWEEN GRADUATION MARKS AND GLASS

The gray graduation marks contrast poorly against the glass syringe's reservoir. Specifically, the markings and background surface have an estimated contrast ratio of 2:1, whereas contrast affording good legibility is in the range of 5:1 to 7:1 (Figure 12.71).*

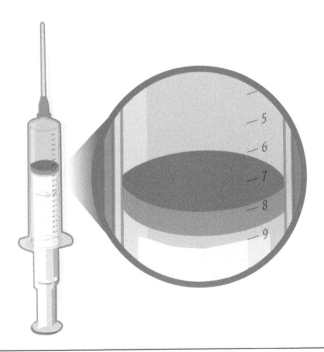

FIGURE 12.71   The gray graduation marks are difficult to read due to the low contrast between the marks and the syringe's reservoir.

---

* According to the World Wide Web Consortium's "Web Content Accessibility Guidelines 2.0," a contrast ratio of at least 5:1 to 7:1 will ensure good legibility of text. Available at http://www.w3.org/TR/WCAG20/

Root Cause #2

SMALL NUMERICAL LABELS

The syringe graduations are labeled with 4-point numerals. When viewed at a distance of 12 inches, numerals of this size subtend a visual angle of 15 arc minutes, which is less than the minimum, recommended visual angle of 16 arc minutes that is necessary to achieve marginally acceptable legibility.[*] As such, the numerals' small size contributed to the reading error (Figure 12.72).

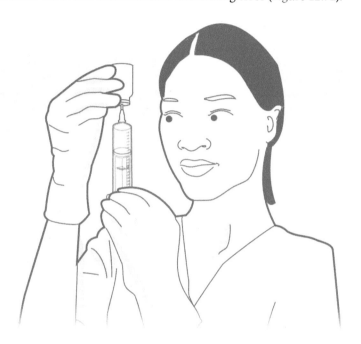

FIGURE 12.72 The graduation numerals are difficult to read due to their small size.

Suggested Mitigation

INCREASE SIZE AND CONTRAST OF MARKINGS AND LABELS

Print higher contrast, darker text[†] markings and associated labels on the syringe barrel. Also, make them somewhat larger, further increasing their legibility (Figure 12.73).

---

[*] ANSI/AAMI HE75:2009/(R)2013, Section 6.2.2.5, "Visual Angle." The standard indicates that the minimum marginally acceptable visual angle is 16 arc minutes.

[†] ANSI/AAMI HE75:2009/(R)2013, Section 10.4.4.2, "Contrast." The standard specifies that a light background with dark text helps maximize readability and legibility.

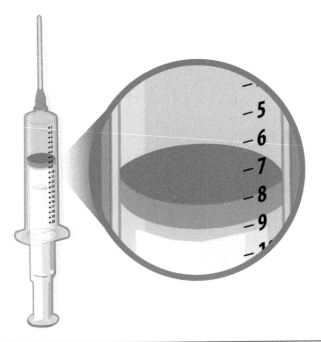

FIGURE 12.73 The larger, bold graduation marks on the revised syringe are more legible.

Product

Electrosurgical Generator and Handpiece

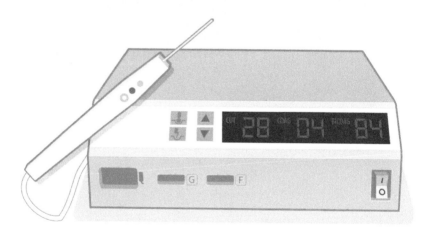

FIGURE 12.74   An electrosurgical generator and handpiece.

An electrosurgical generator and associated controllers (e.g., handpieces foot pedals) are used to cut and coagulate tissue during surgery (Figure 12.74). A system typically includes a base unit that generates the electrical energy from normal AC current and delivers it to the point of tissue application at a selected power level. Different handpieces serve to deliver different forms of energy (e.g., monopolar and bipolar) to produce various effects. Energy flow may be controlled by pressing buttons on a handpiece or by stepping on a foot pedal. The handpiece's primary users are surgeons, but a nurse would gather the packaged handpiece for use during a surgical case.

Use Error
DAMAGE TO SURGICAL FIELD

The circulating nurse retrieved the package containing the electrosurgical generator's handpiece for use during the surgical case. When attempting to open the handpiece's package, the nurse participant pulled with increasing force on the package's pull tab until the package cover suddenly opened widely. The cover's sudden release caused the handpiece to fly into the air and land on the surgical field, potentially injuring the patient.

During the post-test interview, the nurse said, "I just kept pulling harder and harder because it wasn't coming open. Then, before I had a chance to let up, the whole thing ripped apart and the handpiece flew out."

Potential harms
+ Infection
+ Minor tissue injury

Root Cause #1
PULL-TAB FORCE PROFILE

The pull-tab requires a relatively high force (approximately 8 lb) to result in the cover starting to peel away from the underlying tray. Once the cover starts to release, it takes substantially less force to peel it back. The sudden and dramatic reduction in resistance force destabilized the nurse's grip on the package, resulting in the handpiece flying out of the packaging (Figure 12.75).

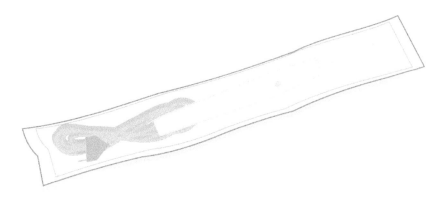

FIGURE 12.75   The user must apply substantial force to begin peeling the cover away from the tray.

Suggested Mitigation

REVISE PULL-TAB'S FORCE PROFILE

Revise the pull-tab's adhesive characteristics so that the tray cover pulls away when applying a moderate, steady force.

Product

Large Volume Infusion Pump

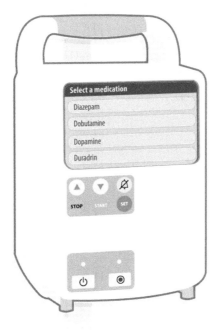

FIGURE 12.76   A large volume infusion pump.

A large volume infusion pump delivers fluids to a patient via an intravenous access (i.e., a needle or catheter placed through the skin and into a vein) (Figure 12.76). The most common user is a nurse who has received in-service training to operate the pump. Anesthesiologists and paramedics might also operate the device, but they might not have received training on its use. Common user tasks include passing an IV bag's tubing through the pump to control flow rate, programming the pump to deliver a prescribed therapy, starting the pump, intermittently monitoring the infusion, responding to any alarms, and disconnecting the patient when the therapy is complete.

Use Error

SELECTED WRONG DRUG FROM DRUG LIBRARY

One test participant selected Dobutamine instead of Dopamine from the list of drugs in the drug library. The participant commented, "I thought I selected Dopamine and then didn't pay much more attention to the drug name while finishing the programming task. I think I checked it once and somehow read 'Dopamine' when I guess it said 'Dobutamine.'"

Potential harms
+ Ineffective therapy
+ Side effects from delivery of incorrect drug

Root Cause #1

SIMILAR DRUG NAME

The drug names Dopamine and Dobutamine are similar in sound and appearance. Both drug names start with "Do," end in "mine" and are about the same length, increasing the chance of selection error (Figure 12.77).

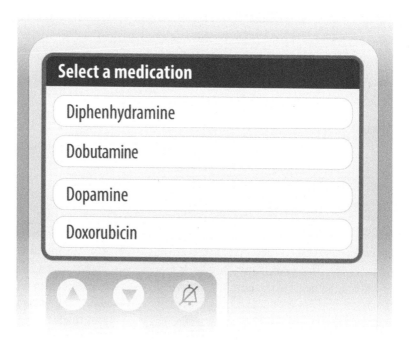

FIGURE 12.77   The two drug names are relatively similar.

Suggested Mitigation

USE TALLMAN LETTERS

Recognizing that drug names themselves cannot be changed, implement a TALLman labeling scheme,* such that the drug names appear as DOBUTamine and DOPamine (Figure 12.78).

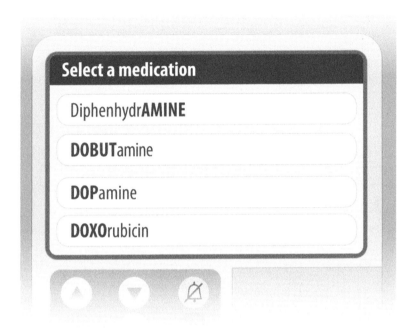

FIGURE 12.78   Presenting drug names using TALLman letters draws attention to the differences among names.

---

* A TALLman labeling scheme calls for capitalizing key letter sequences in a manner that helps differentiate similar drug names. Institute for Safe Medication Practices, "FDA and ISMP Lists of Look-Alike Drug Names with Recommended Tall Man Letters." Available at https://www.ismp.org/tools/tallmanletters.pdf

Product

Hospital Bed

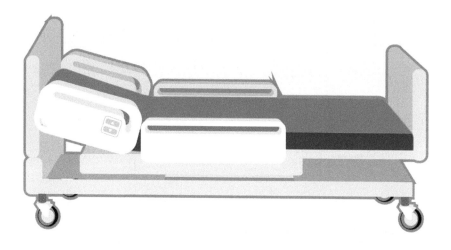

FIGURE 12.79   A hospital bed.

An advanced hospital bed is more than a sleeping surface (Figure 12.79). It serves a wide array of purposes including placing the patient in a specified position (e.g., head-up 30°–45° to help prevent pneumonia), delivering percussive therapy to loosen lung secretions, weighing a patient at risk of dramatic weight loss during a hospital stay, and alerting care unit personnel if the patient awakes and attempts to exit the bed. The beds also provide patients with control over the mattress contour, room radio, television, and room lighting. Some bed functions are accessible only to healthcare professionals because the control panels are outboard—facing away from the patient where they are out of the patient's normal reach. Patients may have significant mental and physical limitations associated with their medical conditions. Sometimes, the patient's visitors might also interact with a bed to assist the patient or perhaps because they are curious about how it works.

Use Error

DID NOT RAISE HEAD OF BED TO 30° ANGLE

In a summative usability test of a hospital bed, participants were required to put the bed into "ventilated patient" therapy mode and adjust the bed angle for a patient on a mechanical ventilator. Three participants did not place the head of bed at the 30° angle indicated for these types of patients. Rather, these participants left the head of bed in a flat (i.e., horizontal) or nearly flat position. One participant commented, "I forgot that last step. I could have used a reminder. Maybe a beep telling me to do it." Another participant commented, "I thought I raised the head of bed, but not enough I guess. I thought it was up enough." A third participant explained, "That's not something that we do on our unit."

Potential harms

✦ Pneumonia

Root Cause #1

INCONSPICUOUS ANGLE INDICATOR

The bed angle indicator is relatively small, and its beige color blends in with the tan head rail, thereby making it relatively inconspicuous. Consequently, some users will likely overlook it. The angle indicator does not serve as an effective visual reminder to place the head of the bed at the prescribed angle for patients on a ventilator (Figure 12.80).

Root Cause #2

LACK OF ACTIVE ALERT

The hospital bed does not actively alert the user when the head of bed is placed at an angle of less than 30° when it is in the "ventilated patient" therapy mode. In other words, it does not draw the user's attention with an additional, salient stimuli, such as a flashing light or a beep.

Suggested Mitigations

ENLARGE AND VISUALLY DISTINGUISH THE BED ANGLE INDICATOR

To make the angle indicator more conspicuous and therefore more likely to remind users to place the head of the bed at the correct angle, enlarge the indicator and use color to distinguish it visually from the beige head rail (Figure 12.81).

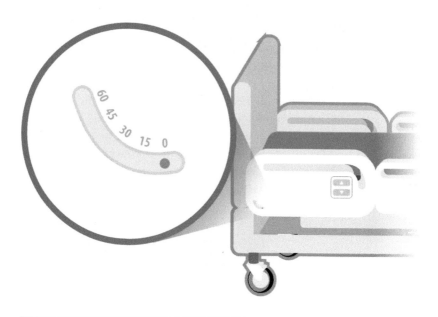

FIGURE 12.80 The bed angle indicator is prone to oversight because it is relatively inconspicuous.

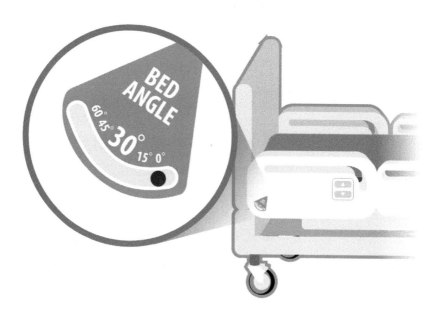

FIGURE 12.81 The revised indicator is larger and brightly colored.

ADD AUDIBLE ALARM

An alarm should sound when the head of the bed is not placed at a 30° or greater angle. Such an alarm would be activated only when the hospital bed is in a particular therapy mode, such as "ventilated patient."

Product

Pen-Injector

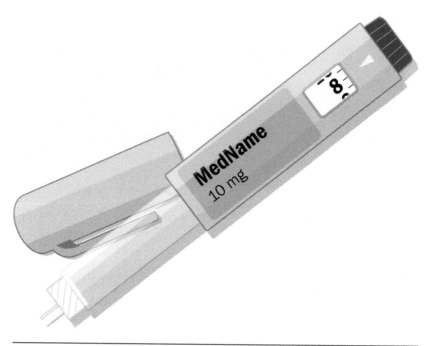

FIGURE 12.82   A pen-injector.

A pen-injector is a drug delivery device designed to deliver a selected dose of a particular drug (Figure 12.82). Although some pen-injectors are used by clinicians, most are used by laypersons who were likely trained to use them properly. After using an adjustment mechanism (e.g., rotary dial) to set a dose, the user presses the pen-injector against a body part (e.g., abdomen, buttocks) and actuates the injection, which usually means pressing a button. Laypersons might have various medical conditions associated with the injection therapy, such as rheumatoid arthritis, that could pose an array of physical and mental limitations to device handling.

Use Error

PREMATURELY WITHDREW NEEDLE FROM SKIN

Three participants withdrew the pen-injector's needle from the injection site before the prescribed 10-second hold-time had elapsed. One participant withdrew the needle immediately after hearing a "click" and commented, "You hear the 'click,' which tells you that the injection is over and you want to get the needle out of you as soon as possible."

The other two participants kept the needle in the injection site for approximately two seconds. One of these participants said, "I don't think the instructions said anything about holding the needle in for a while after pressing the button." Another participant said, "I read the instruction to keep it in for 10 seconds, but figured it was a waste of time. I've been using similar pen-injectors for years. I don't hold them in and have never had a problem. So, I don't see the point. I wouldn't do it at home so I didn't do it here."

Potential harms
  ✦ Underdose

Root Cause #1
MISLEADING AUDITORY FEEDBACK

The pen-injector makes a distinct and brief audible "click" once the medication has been fully ejected from the needle but not yet absorbed into the skin. This sound is the by-product of the internal mechanism's dynamics and seemed to lead one of the participants to withdraw the needle from the injection site almost immediately after hearing the "click" and to mistakenly conclude that the injection was complete even though 10 seconds had not passed (Figure 12.83).

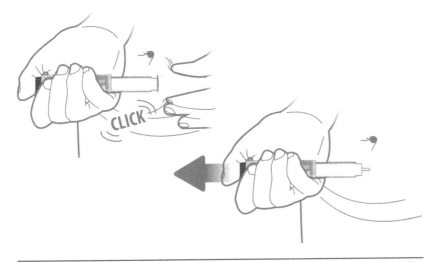

FIGURE 12.83   One participant removed the pen injector from the skin immediately after hearing the "click."

Root Cause #2

SINGLE-MODALITY INSTRUCTIONS

The pen-injector's IFU directs users to keep the device's needle in the injection site for 10 seconds after the device has fully delivered the dose, specifically so that the medication can infuse properly into the injection site rather than ooze out (resulting in an underdose). However, the IFU presents this information as text only, rather than reinforcing the text with an informative graphic. The absence of the graphic reinforcement seemed to contribute to the test participants' lack of awareness of the need to keep the needle in 10 seconds after the click (Figure 12.84).

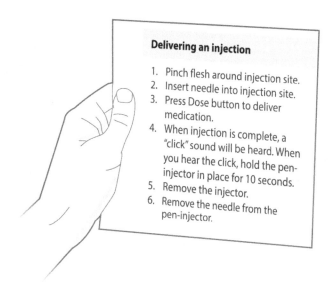

Delivering an injection

1. Pinch flesh around injection site.
2. Insert needle into injection site.
3. Press Dose button to deliver medication.
4. When injection is complete, a "click" sound will be heard. When you hear the click, hold the pen-injector in place for 10 seconds.
5. Remove the injector.
6. Remove the needle from the pen-injector.

FIGURE 12.84   The IFU includes only text instructions.

Root Cause #3

NO STATEMENT OF CONSEQUENCE

The IFU does not explain the consequence of holding the needle in the skin for less than 10 seconds. As a result, one participant chose not to comply with this instruction because she was unaware that holding the needle in place for 10 seconds was necessary to ensure that she received the full dose.

Suggested Mitigations
PROVIDE AUDIBLE FEEDBACK

Redesign the pen-injector to produce an "end of dose delivery" sound at the point in time that the pen-injector should be removed from the injection site. This stimulus could also be augmented by a signal indicating progress such as a ticking noise.

ADD GRAPHICAL INSTRUCTION

Add a graphic to the IFU indicating that the needle should stay in the injection site for 10 seconds after the click to increase the likelihood users hold the pen-injector in place long enough for the injected fluid to infuse properly (Figure 12.85).

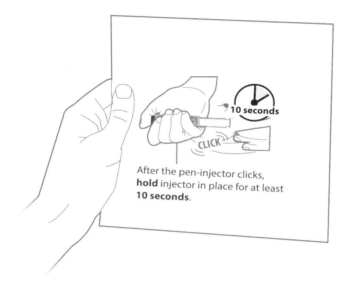

FIGURE 12.85   The new IFU graphic illustrates that the needle should stay in the injection site for 10 seconds.

Product

Blood Gas Analyzer

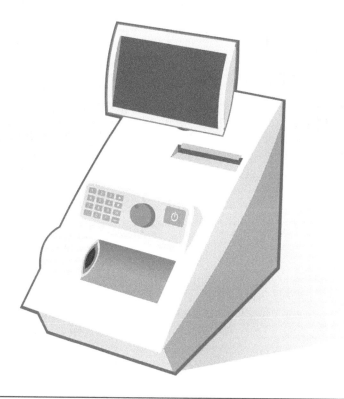

FIGURE 12.86   A blood gas analyzer.

A blood gas analyzer aspirates blood from a syringe and measures pH and the partial pressures of oxygen and carbon dioxide (Figure 12.86). Devices used in hospitals near the point of patient care are likely to be operated by nurses who received in-service training. An analyzer might also be used in a central laboratory, operated by a trained biotechnologist. Typically, the devices sit on a countertop. Maintenance tasks might include calibrating sensors and checking or refilling/replacing reagent supplies—the chemicals necessary to run blood tests. Individual sample tests call upon users to uniquely identify and load the sample, select the desired test (if there are options), dispose of testing by-products (if necessary), and review and process test results.

Use Error
POWERED OFF THE DEVICE

After answering a simulated page (i.e., planned distraction), the participant returned to the analyzer and noticed the screen had turned off. The participant attempted to "wake up" the analyzer from "sleep" mode by pressing the power button, rather than touching the screen. Consequently, the participant powered off the analyzer. Powering off the analyzer aborted the blood test mid-analysis, resulting in a failed test.

The participant reported the following: "I figured that any one of the device's buttons would wake it up. I tried a bunch of the control panel hardware buttons and then figured I would try pressing the power button. I think pressing the power button should wake it up rather than turn it off. My computer works that way. It doesn't feel natural to wake it up by touching a screen that looks dead."

Potential harms
+ Delay in diagnosis

Root Cause #1
HIDDEN FUNCTION

The touch screen-equipped analyzer lacks an indication regarding how to activate the screen when it is in power-saving, "sleep" mode. Not realizing that she had to touch the screen to exit "sleep" mode, the participant erroneously concluded that a button press was required.

Root Cause #2
NEGATIVE TRANSFER

Other devices, such as laptop computers, enable the user to wake the device from sleep mode by pressing the power button. Consequently, the participant incorrectly assumed that the blood analyzer functioned similarly.

Suggested Mitigation
CHANGE RESPONSE TO BUTTON PRESS

Reactivate the screen if the device is in "sleep" mode and the user momentarily presses the power button (Figure 12.87).

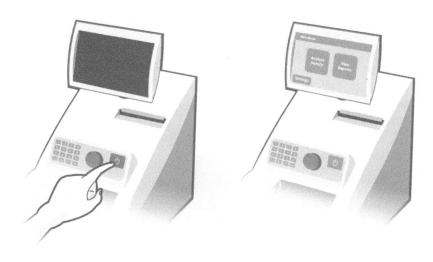

FIGURE 12.87   The revised design enables the user to reactivate the device by momentarily pressing the power button.

Product
Dialysis Solution Bag

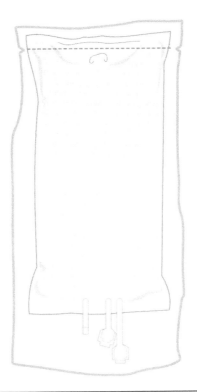

FIGURE 12.88   A dialysis solution bag.

Peritoneal dialysis is a treatment for patients with end-stage renal disease (ESRD) (Figure 12.88). A peritoneal dialysis machine introduces dialysis solution into the abdominal cavity via a catheter. The dialysis solution pulls waste products and excess fluid from the blood, across the peritoneum, and into the abdominal cavity. Subsequently, dialysis solution, along with the waste products and excess fluid, is drained from the abdominal cavity. Dialysis solution bags may be handled by a dialysis nurse or dialysis technician as well as by patients who deliver their own treatment at home. Patients may be experiencing various physical and mental impairments related to their disease, including a degree of "mental fogginess" just before and after treatment.

Use Error

TORE SOLUTION BAG

One participant tore the dialysis solution bag when she opened the bag's overwrap (i.e., outer plastic packaging). When the participant grasped the overwrap's tear strip, she unintentionally grasped the dialysis solution bag as well. Consequently, when she tore open the overwrap, she also tore open the dialysis bag, thereby spilling solution directly onto herself.

The participant said, "I didn't realize I was also pulling on the solution bag when I ripped open the outer bag. I'm surprised the bag isn't more durable. I wouldn't expect that I could also tear it open so easily" (Figure 12.89).

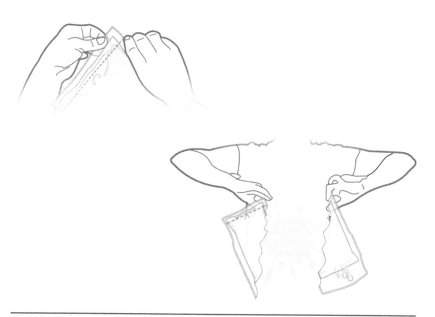

FIGURE 12.89 The participant tore the solution bag and spilled solution onto herself.

Potential harms
- ✦ User discomfort
- ✦ Wasted dialysis solution

Root Cause #1

WEAK BAG MATERIAL

The dialysis solution bag's material is relatively weak, causing the bag to tear relatively easily.

Root Cause #2
INSUFFICIENT OVERWRAP GRIP POINT

Users may grip the packaged solution bag in a manner that physically captures the solution bag between the two sides of the overwrap's tear strip. Consequently, when the participant tore open the overwrap, she also tore open the dialysis solution bag.

Suggested Mitigations
REVISE GRIP POINT

Redesign the overwrap such that the overwrap includes one or more large grip points by which the user can grasp the overwrap without also capturing the solution bag between the overwrap's two sides. For example, consider sealing the overwrap's corners, thereby enabling the user to grasp the overwrap's corner without also grasping (and, therefore, pulling on) the solution bag (Figure 12.90).

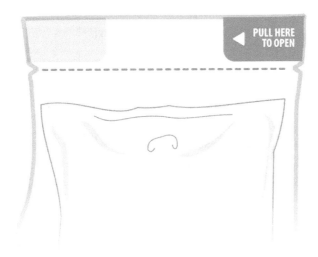

FIGURE 12.90   The redesigned overwrap includes larger grip points.

INCREASE BAG'S DURABILITY

Increase the dialysis bag's strength so that it is less prone to tearing.

Product

Ultrasound Scanner

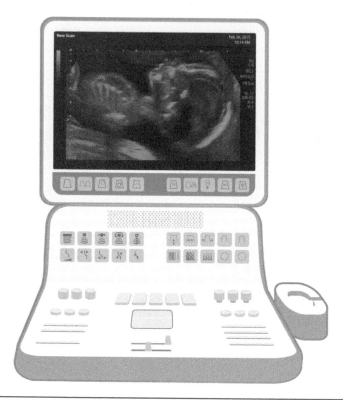

FIGURE 12.91   An ultrasound scanner.

An ultrasound scanner is a diagnostic imaging tool used to visualize internal body structures (Figure 12.91). The device's classic form is a workstation that presents the large display, many controls, and several wands necessary to perform the scanning procedure, although compact, hand-carried devices are becoming common. The device's primary operators are sonographers, who receive extensive training in ultrasound techniques. Sonographers must be certified in some countries. Common user tasks include setting up the device to perform a scan, including entering patient information into on-screen data fields, selecting and connecting a wand to the device, and using the device to take measurements during a scan.

Use Error

PERFORMED INACCURATE MASS TRACE

Two participants traced a mass (i.e., suspected tumor) inaccurately using the ultrasound scanner's touch screen trace tool. One participant made six attempts to create an accurate trace (i.e., outline) and the other participant made five attempts. On the final traces, one participant cut off the lower edge of the mass and the other participant drew a trace that extended well beyond the left edge of the mass.

One participant said, "The line wasn't keeping up with my finger, which was irritating. I couldn't get the trace to align with the mass's edges." The other participant commented, "The touch screen didn't always react when I touched it. I kept trying to move the trace, and sometimes nothing would happen, whereas other times it worked as I expected."

Potential harms

✦ Incorrect diagnosis

Root Cause #1

DELAYED TRACE PRESENTATION

The trace line lags behind a user's finger motions by approximately 0.5 seconds. Consequently, the participants could not immediately see the results of their inputs, which led them to trace the mass inaccurately.

Root Cause #2

INSUFFICIENT TOUCH SCREEN SENSITIVITY

The touch screen has relatively low sensitivity to the user's touch. When these participants attempted to adjust (e.g., resize, shift) the trace, the touch screen did not always react to their touch. Consequently, they could not adjust the trace with sufficient precision to trace the mass accurately (Figure 12.92).

Suggested Mitigation

DECREASE TRACE DELAY

Minimize the lag time between user inputs and display responses associated with drawing a trace.

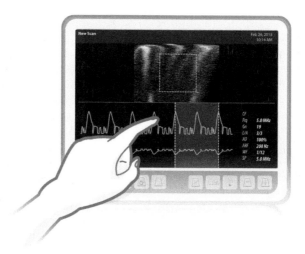

FIGURE 12.92   Participants had difficulty tracing the mass because the touch screen did not always react to their touch.

Suggested Mitigation

PROVIDE ALTERNATIVE POINTING DEVICE

Provide users with the option of a more precise pointing device (e.g., stylus, trackball, mouse) to use in place of using their fingers to draw a trace.

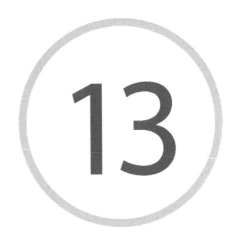

Guide to Designing an Error-Resistant User Interface

INTRODUCTION

In Chapter 10, we discussed user interface design flaws that can lead to use error. Now, to promote user interfaces that are resistant to use error, we offer the following condensed guidance. We derived the guidance from current standards and the lessons we have learned from thousands of usability test sessions and the use errors that have occurred. You could say that we are simply looking at the same issues from opposite perspectives as those in Chapter 10, but we think that this presentation can serve as a helpful checklist of sorts for user interface designers.

Our guidance covers the trinity of user interactions with medical devices—namely, perceptions (P), cognitive processes (C), and actions (A), which are the focus of the kind of "PCA" analysis that regulators have promoted as an effective way to identify potential use errors (see Chapter 6).

Noting that we could fill an entire book with user interface design guidance, we have limited ourselves to providing a constrained set of guidance items that we think will have a disproportionately large benefit in preventing use errors. This approach aligns well with our observation that a large proportion of use errors occurring in usability tests are due to a limited set of common user interface design shortcomings.

PERCEPTIONS

TEXT LEGIBILITY

People will struggle to decipher poorly designed text. Text legibility depends largely on text font, size, and contrast against its background.

+ Text should not be overstyled, if styled at all. Sans serif font—one lacking "flourishes" intended to make letters flow together or simply be decorative—is generally considered to be best. Text should not be overly expanded or condensed in either the vertical or horizontal direction or be constructed with overly thick or thin lines.

+ Text should be large enough for the intended users, who in some cases might have reduced visual acuity, to read it with ease. An FDA guide, "Write It Right,'" suggests using ≥12-point characters to account for vision problems. Meanwhile, ANSI/AAMI HE75:2009/(R)2013[†] suggests using text that subtends a visual angle of at least 16 minutes of arc, with 22–24 minutes of arc being preferable. To determine the visual angle, you can use this formula:

$$a = 3438 \times h/d$$

d = distance between the user's eye and text
h = character height (capital letter height plus the height of a descender, such as the bottom part of the letter "g")[‡] (Figure 13.1)
a = visual angle (measure in minutes, with 60 minutes equaling 1°)
(To convert to degrees, multiply by 360.)

---

[*] Backinger, C. L., and Kingsley, P. A. 1993. "Write It Right: Recommendations for Developing User Instructions for Medical Devices Used in Home Health Care." HHS Publication FDA 93-4258. Available at http://www.fda.gov/downloads/MedicalDevices/DeviceRegulationandGuidance/GuidanceDocuments/UCM070771.pdf.

[†] ANSI/AAMI HE75:2009/(R)2013. "Human Factors Engineering—Design of Medical Devices."

[‡] Arditi, A., and Cho, J. 2007. "Letter Case and Text Legibility in Normal and Low Vision." *Vision Research* 47(19): 2499–2505. Available at http://www.sciencedirect.com/science/article/pii/S0042698907002830

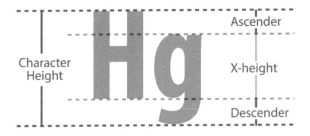

FIGURE 13.1 Character height includes capital letter height and descender height.

EXAMPLE

d = standard viewing distance for reading a book* = 16 inches
× = desired visual angle of 24 minutes of arc (0.0666°)
24 minutes of arc = 3438 × (h ÷ 16 inches)
h = (24 × 16 inches) ÷ 3438 = 0.112 inches = 8-point font

Note: 1 point = 1/72 of an inch (Figure 13.2)

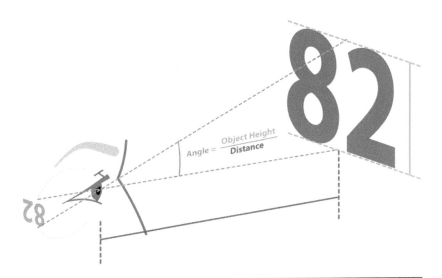

FIGURE 13.2 Visual angle calculation parameters.

* Legge, G., and Bigelow, C. 2011. "Does Print Size Matter for Reading? A Review of Findings from Vision Science and Typography." *Journal of Vision* 11(5): 8. Available at http://jov. arvojournals.org/article.aspx?articleid=2191906

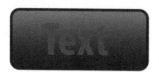 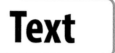

FIGURE 13.3   Poorly contrasted text (left) and well-contrasted text (right).

✦ Text and its background should contrast sharply so that readers can discriminate the letterforms. Black or dark-colored letters contrast very well with white or light backgrounds. Reverse combinations of the same pairs also contrast well. Colors that have a medium value (that are neither light nor dark) contrast poorly with each other (Figure 13.3).

TEXT READABILITY

People may pass over text that looks like too much work to read. They can also be turned off by text that is oddly arranged. These observations apply both to printed and onscreen text, such as text found in user manuals and software prompts, respectively.

✦ Number procedural steps to distinguish the content from other kinds of information and to help users keep their place in an operational sequence.

✦ Avoid splitting critically related information over two pages. For example, avoid separating (1) a series of procedural steps that must performed in rapid sequence or (2) a procedural step and an associated warning.

✦ Separate functionally related groups of information with blank space, thereby emphasizing the groupings and limiting overall information density.

✦ Apply consistent composition rules so that similar information has a similar appearance and may be found in the same general locations on a page or screen.

TEXT CONSPICUITY

People may overlook poorly positioned and formatted text. Drawing their attention depends on the ability to make key information stand out from presumably less important information.

✦ To prevent important text from being overlooked, the text should be sufficiently large to be read quickly and accurately and may be high-lighted (e.g., bolded, colored).

✦ Text is likely to stand out better when it is surrounded by extra blank space—what document designers and typographers call "padding" and "gutters."

✦ To be noticed, text should be placed in view, as opposed to located on an area of a medical device that might not be directly in view (e.g., the back panel).

ALARM DETECTION

✦ Sound-producing devices (e.g., piezoelectric emitters, speakers) should be able to generate sounds that are louder by a selected mar-gin (e.g., 10 dB) than the ambient noise in the use environment.

✦ Tones should not exceed a selected level (e.g., 2000 Hz) because peo-ple with high-frequency hearing loss (i.e., age-related presbycusis*) might not hear them (Figure 13.4).

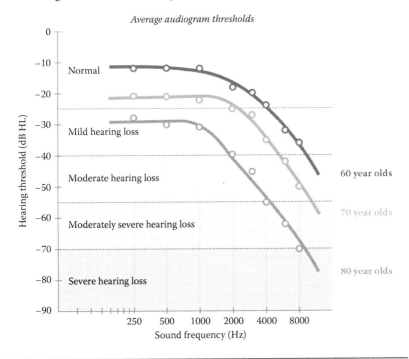

FIGURE 13.4   Average audiogram thresholds for individuals with normal hearing and varying degrees of hearing loss.

---

* As described in ANSI/AAMI HE75:2009/(R)2013, presbycusis is typified by the decreased abil-ity to hear sounds above 2000 Hz, which is common among males in their early 50s and older.

✦ Soundscape designers should use a limited set of tones to convey critical information (e.g., medium- and high-priority alarms) because, with some exceptions, people are not particularly good at making or remembering the associations between tones and assigned meanings.*

Pushbutton Feedback

✦ People like the feel and sensory feedback produced by buttons (excepting on-screen touch targets) that move (i.e., travel) when pressed, clearly communicating when actuation occurs by producing an audible and/or physical "click," for example. This feedback prevents users from pressing a button twice because they are unsure if the first button press registered. It will also prevent cases in which the user thinks the button press registered and it did not.

✦ To make up for the lack of tactile feedback, touch screen targets (also called buttons) should visually react when touched and, in some cases, when released. To give the user a chance to avert an input error due to touching the wrong spot, actuation should occur when the user lifts his or her finger off the button. This gives the user the opportunity to deselect an incorrect target by sliding his or her finger off a target. Users also appreciate when virtual buttons produce audible feedback, such as an electronically produced "click."

Component Visibility

✦ Illuminate elements of a medical device that might be used in dim lighting conditions, such as (1) during a minimally invasive surgical procedure when the operating room lights are dimmed or turned off or (2) when a user operates a blood glucose meter in a dimly lit restaurant. Lighting solutions include spotlighting a specific component, such as a test strip port on a glucose meter, or backlighting a keypad (Figure 13.5).

COGNITION

Mental Calculations

✦ Devices should limit or eliminate the need for users to perform mental calculations or to resort to using a calculator to determine a value. For example, one can design an infusion device to automatically

---

* ANSI/AAMI HE75:2009/(R)2013. Alarm Design, 15.4.8.1 "Inherently Meaningful versus Abstract Auditory Alarm Signals."

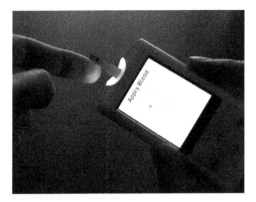

FIGURE 13.5   A glucose meter capable of illuminating the test strip and user's fingertip to facilitate users depositing blood droplets properly in dim lighting conditions.

calculate a total dose based on a flow rate and delivery duration. Some devices even include a built-in virtual calculator for general use.

UNIT CONVERSION

✦ People are prone to err when converting values from one unit of measure to another. Therefore, try to present data in the users' preferred units of measure. Otherwise, give users the option to have the software perform the conversion upon request. This step can help prevent use errors, such as incorrectly converting a newborn baby's weight from pounds to kilograms (Figure 13.6).

INFORMATION RECALL

✦ Medical devices should limit the degree to which users must recall information, such as a lengthy series of procedural steps, product codes, and standard values. Rather, provide job aids, such as Quick

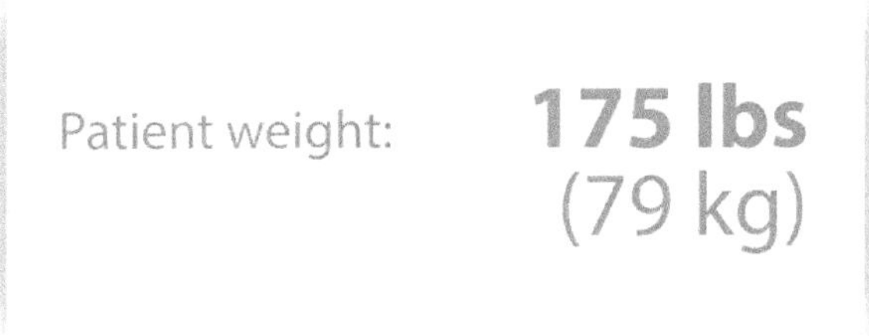

Patient weight: **175 lbs**
(79 kg)

FIGURE 13.6   Parameter displayed in pounds and kilograms.

Reference Guides, a picklist of options, and default values. These job aids can help to make sure that users perform the steps necessary to use a device safely and effectively, such as priming a fluid line before attaching it to a patient's intravenous access.

✦ Where possible, guide users through lengthy procedures and alert them to erroneous actions (e.g., skipping a step, entering an inappropriate value). This can help to keep all types of users, but particularly new users, on track with the correct operational sequence.

ACTION

DEVICE ORIENTATION

✦ Devices should provide definitive cues regarding their proper orientation, thereby preventing people from holding them wrong, or perhaps trying to assemble their myriad components incorrectly. Orientation cues include similarly colored elements that should be aligned, alignment marks such as opposing arrowheads, labels (e.g., "THIS SIDE UP"), and built-in grips that suggest the proper way to hold a component. These cues can help users assemble devices, such as a nebulizer that has multiple components, correctly and more quickly (Figure 13.7).

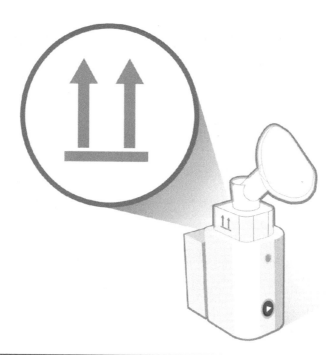

FIGURE 13.7   Symbol indicating proper orientation (i.e., "THIS SIDE UP").

✦ Eliminate features that, by virtue of their appearance, can mislead people. One such example is a pen-injector tip with one end that affords (i.e., suggests) pushing because it looks like a pushbutton on a ballpoint pen, but actually is where the needle pops out.

"Undo" Control

✦ Recognizing that people are prone to error, give them a chance to correct errors before there is a significant consequence. In a software application, an "undo" control gives users the chance to correct a mistake, presuming that the erroneous action is reversible.

Data Entry

✦ Provide users with an example of the proper format for data entry (e.g., "MM/DD/YYYY"). A example will help prevent incorrect entries, such as dates of birth with the month and days switched.

Protection against Inadvertent Actuation

✦ Devices subject to rough handling may be particularly vulnerable to inadvertent control actuation, such as banging an elbow against a control panel. Such events can be prevented by physical guards (e.g., a clear cover), recessing the control, or requiring a protracted input (e.g., pressing and holding down a button).

Instructional Content and Format

✦ People often disregard instructions that may contain content that is essential to preventing use errors. To draw their attention, put instructions where users are most likely to see them, perhaps even making the user handle them before handling the associated device. This could be accomplished by packing a device underneath the instructions, for example, thereby making users "go through" the instructions.

✦ Provide well-designed, well-written instructions that users will actually find helpful. Otherwise, they might skip reading them because the content does not look particularly important or useful due to its low production value.

✦ Complement concise text with simple, informative graphics. Effective graphics focus on key details and eliminate extraneous information, depict only one major step, and clearly show physical manipulations using unambiguous symbols (e.g., arrows) that are optimally located to avoid misinterpretation. Instructions with these attributes drive users to operate devices correctly without having to make guesses about the right way to do things (Figure 13.8).

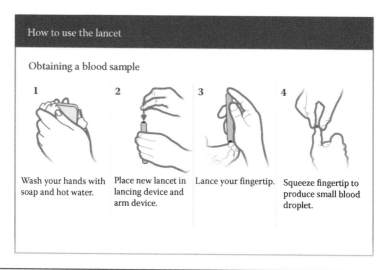

FIGURE 13.8   Graphics complement concise text in this example lancing device's Instructions for Use.

PACKAGE DESIGN

✦ Clearly label a package's contents, emphasizing any differences between it and similar products (e.g., drug delivery devices that contain different drug concentrations). This labeling can prevent users from selecting the wrong item, such as the wrong catheter (e.g., 18 French versus 22 French).

✦ Clearly mark how to open a package properly. This will help prevent people from opening it in a manner (e.g., tearing one end of a sleeve) that damages the contents.

✦ Limit the force required to tear open a package. This will help prevent users from straining themselves and possibly spilling the contents if the package opens abruptly under substantial force.

✦ Ensure that device components, especially small ones, are placed within packages in a manner that prevents them from being overlooked.

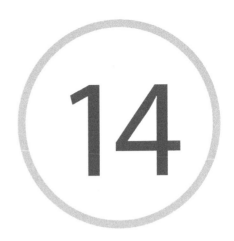

Other Root Cause Analysis Methods

INTRODUCTION

Root cause analysis is a process (aka method or technique) that human factors specialists can approach in a variety of ways. We present our preferred approach in Chapter 2, but there are many other, equally valid processes, tools, and techniques.

This chapter outlines 10 other methods you might consider applying—perhaps as a complement to the one we suggest—when performing a root cause analysis. Some of these tools are broad problem-solving methods (e.g., the five whys, matrix diagrams), whereas others originated from a specific sector, such as aviation (e.g., Human Factors Analysis and Classification System) or healthcare (e.g., UPCARE model). These methods can be used to achieve the same common goal: understand the problem at hand and identify the root causes of the problem.

Do human factors specialists working in the medical device field actually use some of these more formal techniques when they perform root cause analysis? We believe that the people who do are in the minority. That said, a significant proportion of analysts might be applying a thought process that parallels the questioning or diagramming approaches, thereby considering the possible root causes of use error in a systematic manner. Kudos to the analyst or team of them that goes to the length of implementing these methods as a matter of due care.

THE FIVE WHYS

The five whys* is a root cause analysis method used to identify the true or "deepest level" root cause. To apply the method, analysts should ask themselves "why" each time they identify a potential root cause. This approach helps analysts move past symptoms of the problem and ultimately determine the true (i.e., most fundamental) root cause. When the analyst can no longer answer "why," he or she most likely has found the true root cause. Below, we present an example of using the five whys method.

> *Use error:* An emergency responder did not deliver a dose of Naloxone to treat a patient experiencing an opioid overdose.
> *Why #1:* Naloxone did not come out of the syringe when the emergency responder attempted to administer the dose.
> *Why #2:* The emergency responder did not have a functional Naloxone delivery device.
> *Why #3:* The emergency responder did not assemble the Naloxone delivery device correctly.
> *Why #4:* The emergency responder did not know how to attach the vial containing the Naloxone to the syringe.
> *Why #5:* The Instructions for Use did not include all the necessary assembly steps.

The fundamental root cause of this use error is that the instructions do not explain the assembly steps with sufficient detail to guide users, such as the emergency responder in this example, through the assembly process. Consequently, the emergency responder did not assemble the device correctly, and he could not deliver the essential dose of Naloxone to the patient.

Applying this method—asking "why" repeatedly—is the habit of many seasoned human factors specialists who regularly perform root cause analysis.

---

* Andersen, B. and Fagerhaug, T. 2006. *Root Cause Analysis: Simplified Tools and Techniques* (2nd ed.). Milwaukee, WI: ASQ Quality Press.

ISHIKAWA DIAGRAMMING

A problem may arise due to multiple root causes. In such cases, a single root cause alone might not trigger an event. In other words, a problem might not ultimately occur unless all root causes are present in parallel, in a series, or a hybrid of both.

Analysts in other, non-medical industries have employed Ishikawa diagrams (also called fishbone diagrams) to illustrate the relationship between root causes and problems (i.e., effects) (Figure 14.1).

Figure 14.2 depicts categories of root causes of failure in healthcare environments.

Below, we present potential categories for strictly use-related failures that could be presented in an Ishikawa diagram.

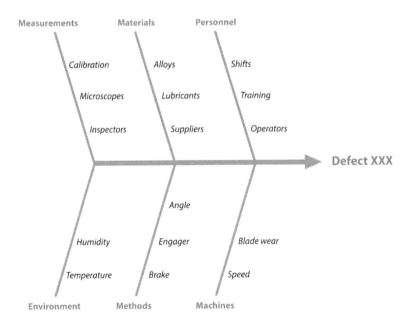

FIGURE 14.1   An example Ishikawa diagram. (Image based on one published by Wikipedia user Daniel Penfield License: http://creativecommons.org/licenses/by-sa/3.0/legalcod. Accessed from http://en.wikipedia.org/wiki/Ishikawa_diagram#mediavièwer/File:Cause_and_effect_diagram_for_defect_XXX.svg)

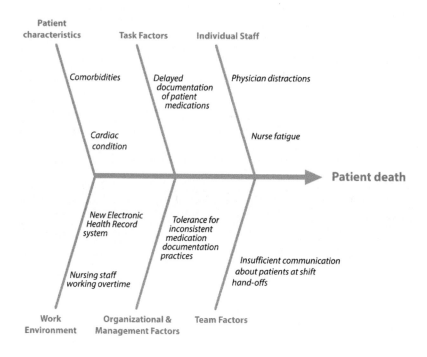

FIGURE 14.2 An example Ishikawa diagram from the healthcare sector.

+ Hardware user interface features (e.g., ergonomics, tactile feedback, arrangement, labeling legibility)
+ Software user interface features (e.g., content, readability, hierarchy prompts)
+ Learning tool features (e.g., format, content availability)
+ Use environment (e.g., equipment, personnel, climate, lighting, noise, architecture distractions)
+ User characteristics (e.g., age, size, strength, education, occupation, knowledge, skills impairments)
+ Training (e.g., amount, format, timing content)

ACCIMAP

An AcciMap illustrates the interrelationship of factors contributing to an accident; a plurality of factors being a defining characteristic of such maps. The technique has been used to illustrate the factors (i.e., root causes) leading to the Challenger Space Shuttle explosion. We present an example in Figure 14.3.

The AcciMap method is particularly effective at showing the cascade of root causes that may result in a dramatic failure (e.g., space shuttle

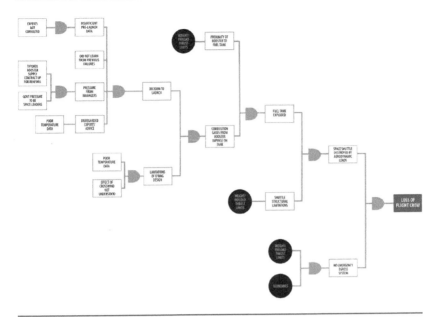

FIGURE 14.3 *Challenger* shuttle AcciMap example.

destruction), as well as root causes as broad-based and seemingly disconnected as workplace cultural and societal influences on the system in play.

Producing such a graphic to depict medical device error might be overkill, noting that a use error does not necessarily constitute a full-blown accident, it might reveal the factors contributing to certain types of use errors and resulting harms. For example, there might be many cascading factors leading to an actual medication delivery error, including the following:

+ Vague hospital policies regarding clinician training to use a given device
+ Limited access to in-service training by part-time workers
+ Specification of excessively wide dosing limits to give clinicians maximum dosing flexibility
+ High ambient noise in the use environment
+ Alarm volume set at low to avoid disturbing patients on a particular care unit
+ User interface design that permits the user to set the high priority alarm volume to low
+ Lack of validation usability testing of pre-production devices by the manufacturer
+ General disdain by the manufacturer for applying human factors engineering in the product development process

Table. Factors That May Lead to Latent Errors	
Type of Factor	**Example**
Institutional/regulatory	A patient on anticoagulants received an intramuscular pneumococcal vaccination, resulting in a hematoma and prolonged hospitalization. The hospital was under regulatory pressure to improve its pneumococcal vaccination rates.
Organizational/management	A nurse detected a medication error, but the physician discouraged her from reporting it.
Work environment	Lacking the appropriate equipment to perform hysteroscopy, operating room staff improvised using equipment from other sets. During the procedure, the patient suffered an air embolism.
Team environment	A surgeon completed an operation despite being informed by a nurse and the anesthesiologist that the suction catheter tip was missing. The tip was subsequently found inside the patient, requiring reoperation.
Staffing	An overworked nurse mistakenly administered insulin instead of an antinausea medication, resulting in hypoglycemic coma.
Task-related	An intern incorrectly calculated the equivalent dose of long-acting MS Contin for a patient who had been receiving Vicodin. The patient experienced an opiate overdose and aspiration pneumonia, resulting in a prolonged ICU course.
Patient characteristics	The parents of a young boy misread the instructions on a bottle of acetaminophen, causing their child to experience liver damage.

FIGURE 14.4 Factors that may lead to latent errors. (Reproduced from AHRQ. "AHRQ Patient Safety Network—Root Cause Analysis." 2014, August 1. Accessed from http://psnet.ahrq.gov/primer.aspx?primerID=10)

The Agency for Healthcare Research and Quality (AHRQ) recognizes that use errors can arise due to root causes that go well beyond user interface flaws. In the table in Figure 14.4, AHRQ provides examples of factors leading to what the agency terms "latent errors." The agency suggests that, once a use error is identified, a "multidisciplinary team should then analyze the sequence of events leading to the error, with the goal of identifying how the event occurred (through identification of active errors) and why the event occurred (through systematic identification and analysis of latent errors)."[*]

As you can see, an AcciMap fosters a systems-level view of the ultimate use error's root causes. The question is whether this tool could be helpful in a prospective analysis of potential use errors. We believe that it could help in situations in which user interface developers have the opportunity to research systems-level issues that have bearing in the user interface design process. It could also be an effective way to illustrate the multiple root causes of a use error that occurs in a usability test, augmenting narrative descriptions. Alternatively, analysts might choose to sketch such diagrams simply to organize their thoughts about the factors leading to a use error.

---

[*] "AHRQ Patient Safety Network—Root Cause Analysis." August 1, 2014. Accessed from http://psnet.ahrq.gov/primer.aspx?primerID=10

THE JOINT COMMISSION'S FRAMEWORK FOR CONDUCTING A ROOT CAUSE ANALYSIS

In 2013, the Joint Commission published a revised framework for the identification of root causes of a sentinel (i.e., fatal) event.[*] Their framework includes a series of 24 questions, reproduced with permission below that investigators can ask about a given event.

1. What was the intended process flow?
2. Were there any steps in the process that did not occur as intended?
3. What human factors were relevant to the outcome?
4. How did the equipment performance affect the outcome?
5. What controllable environmental factors directly affected this outcome?
6. What uncontrollable external factors influenced this outcome?
7. Were there any other factors that directly influenced this outcome?
8. What are the other areas in the organization where this could happen?
9. Was the staff properly qualified and currently competent for their responsibilities at the time of the event?
10. How did actual staffing compare with ideal levels?
11. What is the plan for dealing with staffing contingencies?
12. Were such contingencies a factor in this event?
13. Did staff performance during the event meet expectations?
14. To what degree was all the necessary information available when needed? Accurate? Complete? Unambiguous?
15. To what degree was the communication among participants adequate for this situation?
16. Was this the appropriate physical environment for the processes being carried out for this situation?
17. What systems are in place to identify environmental risks?
18. What emergency and failure-mode responses have been planned and tested?
19. How does the organization's culture support risk reduction?
20. What are the barriers to communication of potential risk factors?
21. How is the prevention of adverse outcomes communicated as a high priority?
22. How can orientation and in-service training be revised to reduce the risk of such events in the future?

---

[*] The Joint Commission. March 21, 2013. Root Cause Analysis and Action Plan Framework Template. Accessed from http://www.jointcommission.org/framework_for_ conducting_a_root_cause_analysis_and_action_plan/

23.   Was available technology used as intended?

24.   How might technology be introduced or redesigned to reduce risk in the future?

The framework employs a table (what others might call a root cause summary table[*]) that tasks investigators with not only identifying root causes of a given event, but also developing a plan of action to prevent reoccurrences. Notably, the Joint Commission states that the framework could be applied to cases of use error, but that it also applies to cases in which there has not yet been a use error (i.e., prospective analysis).

We see value in the application of a similar framework to the analysis of use errors that occur during a usability test. But, taking this approach, analysts will undoubtedly face limitations regarding their ability to prospectively answer questions about use scenarios with the same degree of certainty that one could have in a retrospective analysis of an actual use error.

SIDEBAR 14.1   DEFINITION OF "SENTINEL EVENT"

The Joint Commission defines the term "sentinel event" as follows: "A sentinel event is an unexpected occurrence involving death or serious physical or psychological injury, or the risk thereof. Serious injury specifically includes loss of limb or function. The phrase 'or the risk thereof' includes any process variation for which a recurrence would carry a significant chance of a serious adverse outcome.

Such events are called 'sentinel' because they signal the need for immediate investigation and response.

The terms 'sentinel event' and 'error' are not synonymous; not all sentinel events occur because of an error, and not all errors result in sentinel events."[*]

---

[*] Sentinel Events. 2013. "Comprehensive Accreditation Manual for Hospitals." Accessed from http://www.jointcommission.org/assets/1/6/CAMH_2012_Update2_24_SE.pdf

---

Here are some sample questions pertaining more specifically to the identification of a medical device's user interface design flaws that could be useful when trying to identify root causes of use errors. Consider it a starting

---

[*] Rooney, J. and Vanden Heuvel, L. July 1, 2004. "Root Cause Analysis for Beginners." Accessed from https://servicelink.pinnacol.com/pinnacol_docs/lp/cdrom_web/safety/management/accident_investigation/Root_Cause.pdf

point for a customized list of questions, potentially including some from the AHRQ set listed before and other sources, that pertain well to the medical device under evaluation:

✦ Did the device exceed the user's reading ability?
✦ Did the device exceed the user's physical ability?
✦ Did the device (or Instructions for Use) communicate using unfamiliar terms?
✦ Was essential information illegible?
✦ Did the device fail to present information in an appropriate, timely manner?
✦ Did the device's Instructions for Use misinform or misdirect the user?
✦ Did the device exceed the user's memory capacity?
✦ Did the device fail to provide sufficient feedback in response to user actions?
✦ Did the device make it difficult for the user to assess its operational status?
✦ Did the device oversaturate the user with information?
✦ Did the device require the user to work too quickly?
✦ Was the device missing an essential guard?
✦ Did the device expose components (e.g., controls) to inadvertent actuation?
✦ Did the device operate in a different manner than a similar device with which the user has prior experience?
✦ Did the device produce a signal (e.g., visual indication, audible tone) that was difficult for the user to detect?
✦ Did the device produce a single modality signal, rather than redundant cues?
✦ Did the device fail to draw the user's attention to critical information?
✦ Did the device lack the means to undo an incorrect action?
✦ Did the device fail to prompt the user to confirm a critical action or change?
✦ Did the device lack the necessary physical, visual, or audible cues to guide users to interact with it properly?
✦ Did the device have any hidden features or functions that the user could overlook or misidentify?
✦ Did a warning or caution message fail to state the consequence of a use error?
✦ Was the training to use the device inadequate?
✦ Is there a mismatch between the device's workflow and the user's mental model?

Here are a few more questions that could help differentiate a use error that is legitimately caused by a user interface design flaw from those that could legitimately be attributed to test artifact, participation in the test by an unqualified test participant, or knowing non-compliance.

+ Was there a test condition that significantly altered the way the user interacted with the device?
+ Did the user knowingly depart from a prescribed approach to using the device in a safe and effective manner?
+ Was the user unqualified to serve as a test participant according to screening criteria or other demographic or experience-related requirements?

UPCARE MODEL

Another root cause analysis framework of sorts, which is keenly focused on the evaluation of medical device error is called the UPCARE model. "The UPCARE model takes its name from its six domain areas: (1) unmet user needs, (2) perception, (3) cognition, (4) actions, (5) results, and (6) evaluation. Each of these areas is broken down into components discovered in the analysis of use errors involving medical devices…'"

The framework (aka model) describes user interface design shortcomings that could lead to use error and then takes the analysis further by specifying results (i.e., harms including injury and death). It also describes the means to learn more about the potential for use error in the real world as well as how to expose use errors in a usability test. The UPCARE model's developers recognize that a comprehensive analysis of accidents (aka adverse outcomes, sentinel events) should also consider broader-based contributing factors such as those considered in the development of an AcciMap (discussed earlier). The framework[†] poses many potential causes of use error, a subset of which is listed verbatim below.

---

* Kaye, R., North, R. A., and Peterson K. M. (2003). "UPCARE: An Analysis, Description and Educational Tool for Medical Device Use Problems," Section 3.1, "Model Description." Accessed from http://www.researchgate.net/publication/237568891_UPCARE_AN_ANALYSIS_DESCRIPTION_AND_EDUCATIONAL_TOOL_FOR_MEDICAL_DEVICE_USE_PROBLEMS

† Kaye, R., North, R. A., and Peterson K. M. (n.d.). "UPCARE: An Analysis, Description and Educational Tool for Medical Device Use Problems," Section 3.1, "Model Description." Accessed from http://www.researchgate.net/publication/237568891_UPCARE_AN_ANALYSIS_DESCRIPTION_AND_EDUCATIONAL_TOOL_FOR_MEDICAL_DEVICE_USE_PROBLEMS

Unmet User Needs

The user needed, but didn't have:

Set-up, configuration, repair

1. Efficient, intuitive set-up and start up procedures
2. Effective cues or instruction for proper device operation
3. Instructions on how to use device under atypical conditions or for specific applications

User-device interaction

1. Indication of current setting or default mode
2. Safe default mode/fail-safe mode
3. Ability to immediately stop device action or process
4. Feedback in response to critical control actions
5. Handy quick-reference material or embedded help
6. Assistance in solving problem or troubleshooting
7. Sufficient device quality to get reasonable results in time allowed
8. Relief from need to "work around" requirements of device use

Monitor and detect normal v. abnormal state (in patient and/or device)

1. Indication of critical change in patient condition
2. Indication that device was operating properly
3. Indication of device failure or critical change in device operation
4. Indication of battery (or charge) end-of-life condition in time to respond

Understanding of device output

1. User unaware of how to correctly interpret clinical meaning of device output (e.g., diagnostic test results)

Perception

User couldn't see device displays, labels, or markings

1. Blocked from view
2. Not bright enough
3. Glare on display
4. Font size too small

User couldn't hear device alarms or audio feedback

1. Volume too low
2. Audio frequency too high or low

User couldn't feel or interpret tactile feedback from device

COGNITION

Information interpretation

1. Text, number, or status indication difficult to visually locate in a complex display
2. Packaging, markings, or displayed data on two or more devices or components appeared similar causing misidentification or confusion
3. Labeling on device or overall device configuration was misleading regarding identity, operation, or use
4. Input, output, level, or calibration values confusing because of unexpected or nonstandard names, abbreviations, or units
5. Navigation through menus or other interface features difficult/confusing

Feedback

1. Difficult or impossible to understand state or mode of device from inadequate, confusing or lack of feedback in response to user actions
2. Misleading feedback or cues provided by device indicated different device or clinical condition than actual

User expectations

1. Expected device operating status or mode to be different than it was
2. Expected device (or component) to operate like similar device previously used due to general appearance/name
3. Expected device-based treatment parameters (e.g., treatment, dose) to be consistent with prior experience
4. Excessive alarms, signals, or emphasis of unimportant information desensitized user to priority of critical information ("nuisance alarms")

Knowing what to do

1. Instructions inadequate to support user while using device
2. User training inadequate

3. Device data insufficient for user to diagnose patient situation—adjust treatment, etc.
4. User does not understand device communication (e.g., error codes, status indication, etc.)
5. User was confused by required sequence of actions for device use

ACTIONS

Set-up

1. Connected components incorrectly
2. Placed, inserted, or secured components incorrectly
3. Assembled components incorrectly

Input and control

1. Unintentionally activated wrong key, button, or other control (e.g., keystroke error)
2. Activated device or component at wrong time or in incorrect sequence
3. Took action to solve problem and caused a future problem (e.g., defeated alarm which allowed unsafe patient condition to go undetected)

Physical damage

1. Walked or bumped into device/component, knocked over, etc.
2. Damaged device while adjusting, moving, or transporting patient
3. Repeated use degrades device interface components (e.g., fingernails scratch surface or break keypad)

RESULTS

To patient

1. Patient injured or died
2. Unnecessary clinical complication

To device user

1. Death or injury of caregiver or bystander
2. Delay in providing treatment
3. Necessity to use less-preferred treatment option
4. Frustration, anxiety for user or healthcare provider team

To device or environment

1.   Device damaged or destroyed

EVALUATION

Collect user-device interaction information

1.   User interviews
2.   Field observations

Analyze context of use error

1.   Task walkthroughs
2.   Task analysis

Test user-device interaction

1.   Usability evaluation

We think that these examples are most relevant to determining the root causes of medical device use error. Below, we describe several additional techniques that can support analysts as they characterize a problem that warrants root cause analysis and/or as they perform root cause analysis. We briefly summarize the methods and suggest that readers reference the listed sources to learn more about how to apply each method.

MATRIX DIAGRAMS

Matrix diagrams enable analysts to compare several possible root causes and determine which root cause contributes most to a set of problems or events. Developing and analyzing a matrix diagram involves the following steps[*]:

1.   Selecting the problem characteristics of interest (e.g., dose set incorrectly, drug not inspected) and possible causes (e.g., illegible text, unclear information in instructions) to be investigated
2.   Creating an appropriately sized matrix, such as a 5×5 square matrix

---

[*] Andersen, B. and Fagerhaug, T. 2006. *Root Cause Analysis: Simplified Tools and Techniques* (2nd ed.). Milwaukee, WI: ASQ Quality Press.

3. Plotting the variables on the matrix
4. Rating the strength of the relationship (e.g., 1 = weak, 5 = medium, 9 = strong) between each problem characteristic and possible cause
5. Calculating the total for each root cause across all problem characteristics
6. Reviewing highly-rated root causes to identify the most likely root cause(s)

CRITICAL DECISION METHOD (CDM)

CDM is used to uncover and understand domain knowledge regarding how subject matter experts make decisions, by interviewing one or more experts. Analysts can employ CDM to understand an expert's cognitive process during an accident, critical cues that may have led to an error, and the factors affecting the expert's decision making process.[*] All of these inputs can then be used to perform root cause analysis of the accident or error.

SYSTEMS-THEORETIC ACCIDENT MODEL AND PROCESSES (STAMP)

STAMP is an accident analysis model that is based on systems theory. In the model, "each level of the sociotechnical structure of a system can be described in terms of levels of control. Each level exercises control over emergent properties, in this case safety, arising from (1) component failures, (2) dysfunctional interactions among components, or (3) unhandled environmental disturbances at a lower level."[†] Accordingly, the model enables analysts to identify root causes in each of these categories.

THE HUMAN FACTORS ANALYSIS AND CLASSIFICATION SYSTEM (HFACS)

HFACS is used to analyze aviation accidents and could be employed to analyze errors in other domains. The method defines four levels at which errors can occur:

1. Unsafe acts
2. Preconditions for unsafe acts

---

[*] Klein, G.A., Calderwood, R., and MacGregor, D. 1989. "Critical Decision Method for Eliciting Knowledge." *IEEE Transactions on Systems, Man, and Cybernetics* 19:3.

[†] Leveson, N. 2004. "A New Accident Model for Engineering Safer Systems." http://sunnyday. mit.edu/accidents/safetyscience-single.pdf

3. Unsafe supervision

4. Organizational influences

A review of these levels can enable analysts to identify and classify the causes of accidents.[*]

EVENT ANALYSIS FOR SYSTEMIC TEAMWORK (EAST)

The EAST method is used to understand how teams collaborate to complete tasks by utilizing analysis tools, such as communication usage diagrams, social network analysis, and CDM. The method helps analysts define who is included in the team for a given scenario, when specific tasks occur, where teammates are positioned, how they collaborate and communicate, what information is used, and what knowledge is shared among teammates.[†]

---

[*] Shappell, S.A. and Wiegmann, D.A. 2000. "The Human Factors Analysis and Classification System—HFACS." Report number DOT/FAA/AM-00/7. Office of Aviation Medicine.

[†] Walker, G.H., Gibson, H., Stanton,. N.A., Baber, C., Salmon, P., and Green, D. 2006. Event analysis of systemic Teamwork (EAST): A novel integration of ergonomics methods to analyse C4i activity. *Ergonomics.* 49:12–13.

Resources

BOOKS

Andersen, B., and Fagerhaug, T. 2006. *Root Cause Analysis: Simplified Tools and Techniques* (2nd ed.). Milwaukee, WI: ASQ Quality Press.

Dekker, S. 2013. *The Field Guide to Understanding Human Error* (2nd ed.). Farnham, UK: Ashgate Publishing.

Dumas, J., and Loring, B. 2008. *Moderating Usability Tests Principles and Practices for Interacting.* Amsterdam: Morgan Kaufmann/Elsevier.

Hallinan, J. 2009. *Why We Make Mistakes.* New York: Broadway Books.

Nielsen, J. 1994. *Usability Inspection Methods.* New York: Wiley.

Norman, D. 1990. *The Design of Everyday Things.* New York: Doubleday Business.

Reason, J. 1990. *Human Error.* Cambridge, England: Cambridge University Press.

Weinger, M., Wiklund, M., and Gardner-Bonneau, D. 2011. *Handbook of Human Factors in Medical Device Design.* Boca Raton, FL: CRC Press.

Wiklund, M., Kendler, J., and Strochlic, A. 2015. *Usability Testing of Medical Devices* (2nd ed.). Boca Raton, FL: CRC Press.

Wiklund, M., and Wilcox, S. 2005. *Designing Usability into Medical Products.* Boca Raton, FL: CRC Press.

ARTICLES AND REPORTS

AAMI TIR50:2014. 2014. "Technical Information Report, Post-Market Surveillance of Use Error Management." Arlington, VA: Association for the Advancement of Medical Instrumentation. Available at http://my.aami.org/store/detail. aspx?id=TIR50-PDF

AHRQ Patient Safety Network—"Root Cause Analysis." August 1, 2014. Available at http://psnet.ahrq.gov/primer.aspx?primerID=10

Hyman, W. 1995, May. "The Issue Is 'Use,' Not 'User,' Error." Medical Device and Diagnostic Industry. Available at http://www.mddionline.com/article/issue-use-not-user-error

Kaye, R., North, R. A., and Peterson K. M. (n.d.). "UPCARE: An Analysis, Description and Educational Tool for Medical Device Use Problems," Section 3.1, "Model Description." Available at http://www.researchgate.net/publication/237568891_UPCARE_AN_ANALYSIS_DESCRIPTION_AND_EDUCATIONAL_TOOL_FOR_MEDICAL_DEVICE_USE_PROBLEMS

Klein, G. A., Calderwood, R., and MacGregor, D. 1989. Critical decision method for eliciting knowledge. *IEEE Transactions on Systems, Man, and Cybernetics* 19:3.

Leveson, N. 2004. "A New Accident Model for Engineering Safer Systems." Available at http://sunnyday.mit.edu/accidents/safetyscience-single.pdf

Rooney, J., and Vanden Heuvel, L. July 1, 2014. "Root Cause Analysis for Beginners." Available at https://servicelink.pinnacol.com/pinnacol_docs/lp/cdrom_web/safety/management/accident_investigation/Root_Cause.pdf

Shappell, S. A., and Wiegmann, D. A. 2000. "The Human Factors Analysis and Classification System—HFACS." Report number DOT/FAA/AM-00/7. Office of Aviation Medicine.

The Joint Commission. March 21, 2013. Root Cause Analysis and Action Plan Framework Template. Accessed from http://www.jointcommission.org/framework_for_conducting_a_root_cause_analysis_and_action_plan/

U.S. FOOD AND DRUG ADMINISTRATION (FDA) PUBLICATIONS

The following FDA human factors-related documents are available on the FDA website:

Backinger, C. L., and Kingsley, P. A. 1993. "Write It Right: Recommendations for Developing User Instructions for Medical Devices Used in Home Health Care." HHS publication FDA 93-4258. Available at http://www.fda.gov/downloads/MedicalDevices/DeviceRegulationandGuidance/GuidanceDocuments/UCM070771.pdf

CFR—Code of Federal Regulations, "Title 21—Food and Drugs," Chapter I—"Food and Drug Administration," Department of Health and Human Services, Subchapter H—"Medical Devices," Part 820, "Quality System Regulation." Available at http://www.accessdata.fda.gov/scripts/cdrh/cfdocs/cfcfr/CFRSearch.cfm?CFRPart=820&showFR=1

"Draft Guidance for Industry and Food and Drug Administration Staff—Applying Human Factors and Usability Engineering to Optimize Medical Device Design." Available at http://www.fda.gov/downloads/MedicalDevices/DeviceRegulationandGuidance/GuidanceDocuments/UCM259760.pdf

"Medical Device Use-Safety: Incorporating Human Factors Engineering into Risk Management." Available at http://www.fda.gov/downloads/MedicalDevices/.../ucm094461.pdf

STANDARDS

ANSI/AAMI HE75:2009/(R)2013. "Human Factors Engineering—Design of Medical Device." Arlington, VA: Association for the Advancement of Medical Instrumentation. Available at http://my.aami.org/store/detail.aspx?id=HE75

IEC 60601-1-6 "Medical Electrical Equipment—Part 1–6: General Requirements for Basic Safety and Essential Performance—Collateral Standard: Usability." Geneva, Switzerland: International Organization for Standardization. Available at http://webstore.iec.ch/Webstore/webstore.nsf/mysearchajax?Openform&key=60601-1-6&sorting=&start=1&onglet=1, publication detail.

IEC 62366-1:2015. 2015. "Medical Devices—Application of Usability Engineering to Medical Devices." Geneva, Switzerland: International Organization for Standardization. Available at https://webstore.iec.ch/publication/21863

ISO 13485:2003. 2003. "Medical Devices—Quality Management Systems—Requirements for Regulatory Purposes." Geneva, Switzerland: International Organization for Standardization. Available at http://www.iso.org/iso/catalogue_detail?csnumber=36786

ISO 14971:2007. 2007. Medical Devices—Application of Risk Management to Medical Devices." Geneva, Switzerland: International Organization for Standardization. Available at http://www.iso.org/iso/catalogue_detail?csnumber=38193

WEBSITES

"Inspections, Compliance, Enforcement, and Criminal Investigations, Corrective and Preventive Actions (CAPA)." Available at http://www.fda.gov/iceci/inspections/inspectionguides/ucm170612.htm

Links to medical devices design and evaluation articles published by one of this book's coauthors (Michael Wiklund) in "Medical Device & Diagnostic Industry." Available at http://www.mddionline.com/search/node/michael%20wiklund

"Medical Devices: Guidance Document, Classification of Medical Devices, MEDDEV 2." 4/1 Rev. June 9, 2010. Available at http://ec.europa.eu/health/medical-devices/files/meddev/2_4_1_rev_9_classification_en.pdf

Medical Device Safety Calendar 2009. Published by FDA. Available at http://www.fda.gov/downloads/MedicalDevices/Safety/AlertsandNotices/UCM134873.pdf

US Food and Drug Administration. (n.d.). Available at http://www.fda.gov/MedicalDevices/DeviceRegulationandGuidance/HumanFactors/ucm124829.htm

Usability-related information with a European perspective. Available at http://www.usabilitynet.org/home.htm

Index

Note: Page numbers followed by "*fn*" indicate footnotes.

A

AAMI, *see* Association for Advancement of Medical Instrumentation (AAMI)
AcciMap method, 220
    AHRQ, 222
    Challenger shuttle AcciMap example, 221
    interrelationship of factors, 220
    latent errors, 222
ACME, 92, 94
Action(s), 229
    data entry, 215
    device orientation, 214–215
    errors, 39, 40
    graphics complement concise text, 216
    instructional content and format, 215
    package design, 216
    protection against inadvertent actuation, 215
    "undo" control, 215
Advanced life support (ALS), 55
Adverse event, *see* Medical device accident
AED, *see* Automated external defibrillator (AED)

Agency for Healthcare Research and Quality (AHRQ), 222
ALAP, *see* As low as possible (ALAP)
Alarms, 69
    detection, 211–212
ALARP, *see* As low as reasonably practicable (ALARP)
ALS, *see* Advanced life support (ALS)
Anecdotal evidence analysis, 10
Anxious, 63
As low as possible (ALAP), 36
As low as reasonably practicable (ALARP), 36
Associated controllers, 184
Association for Advancement of Medical Instrumentation (AAMI), 9, 53
Auto-injector, 148
    auto-injector's inspection window, 149
    increasing inspection window conspicuity, 150
    injecting contaminated drug, 151
    inspect drug, 149
    no explanation of consequence, 150
    revised auto-injector features larger window, 150
    small inspection window, 149
    state consequence of injecting contaminated drug, 150–151